Choosing Autonomy

THE PHYSICIAN'S GUIDE TO RETURNING TO PRIVATE PRACTICE

RANDY BAUMAN

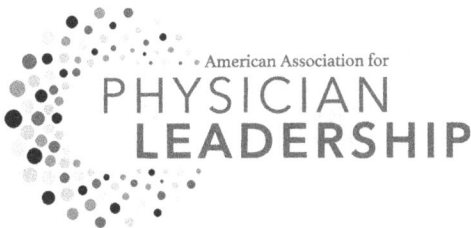

American Association for
PHYSICIAN
LEADERSHIP

AAPL books are available at special quantity discounts to use as premiums and sales promotions, or for use in corporate training programs. For more information, please write to Special Sales at journal@physicianleaders.org

This publication is designed to provide general information and is sold with the understanding that neither the author nor the publisher is engaged in rendering legal, accounting, ethical, or clinical advice. If legal or other expert advice is required, the services of a competent professional person should be sought.

13   8 7 6 5 4 3 2 1

Copyedited, typeset, indexed, and printed in the United States of America

PUBLISHER
Nancy Collins

EDITORIAL ASSISTANT
Jennifer Weiss

DESIGN & LAYOUT
Carter Publishing Studio

COPYEDITOR
Pat George

Table of Contents

Dedication

To my daughter, Arial. May the bright sun and the gift of knowledge coupled with inquisitiveness always shine on you.

Acknowledgements

One of my favorite movies is "Groundhog Day," with Bill Murray playing the TV weatherman stuck in Punxsutawney, Pennsylvania, forced to relive the same day, Groundhog Day, over and over. After a while he has been through the same day so many times he knows virtually everything that is going to happen and when.

In one scene, he predicts a stream of events to his co-star, Andie McDowell, seconds before they happen.

"Is this some kind of trick?" she says.

He replies, "Maybe the real God uses tricks. Maybe He's not omnipotent. Maybe He's just been around so long, He knows everything."

That is exactly how I feel in living through what I call "The Cycle of Physician Employment." I've see this movie before and I wonder if they'll change the ending.

Over the past couple of years, my business partners and I have noticed that an increasing number of the practice valuations we have done were for hospitals selling the practices back to physicians. We also started seeing client engagements helping physician groups extract themselves from hospital employment and return to private practice. On a plane between Las Vegas and Des Moines, the light bulb came on and the idea for this guide was born.

I want to thank my colleagues Arial Simpson and Pat Aubort for their support and input on early drafts.

I want to thank my sweetheart and love of my life, Christine Picior, for her kind and loving support through the days, nights, and weekends I spent writing and re-writing.

I want to thank Patricia George of Greenbranch for her world-class editing skills. I enjoy writing and she makes me look better at it than I am.

Finally I want to thank Nancy Collins and all the great people at Greenbranch Publishing for supporting this book from its earliest idea through what finally emerged.

RANDY BAUMAN
May, 2016

About the Author

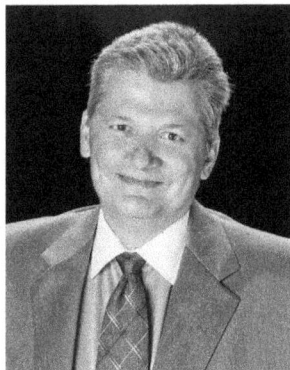

Randy Bauman is president of Delta Health Care (www.deltahealthcare.com) in Franklin, Tennessee. For over 30 years, Randy has advised physician groups and hospitals on the business of physician practice, including hospital/physician network development, group practice development, strategic planning, mergers and acquisitions, group practice formations, physician compensation, governance, operations, and practice valuations.

His books, articles and speeches challenge conventional wisdom and the lemming behavior in healthcare.

He is a frequent speaker at Medical Group Management Association (MGMA) and Healthcare Financial Management Association (HFMA) chapters and other healthcare organizations on a diverse range of topics.

He has been interviewed by and had articles published in numerous healthcare publications, including *The Journal of Medical Practice Management, Medical Economics, The Physician's Advisory, Doctor's Digest, Unique Opportunities, ACP Observer, The Journal of Family Practice,* and *Group Practice Solutions.*

His previous book, *Time to Sell? Guide to Selling a Physician Practice,* was originally published by Greenbranch Publishing in 2008 and was revised in a third edition in 2016. He is a member of the MGMA, the American Health Lawyers Association, and Toastmasters International.

He lives in Mesquite, Nevada, and in his spare time he pursues his passions for travel, photography, and motorcycling. Contact Randy Bauman at rb@deltahealthcare.com.

Introduction

*All marriages are happy. It's the living together afterward
that causes all the trouble.*
RAYMOND HULL

When it comes to physicians being employed by hospitals,
the above quote is more apropos than ever. While many
hospitals continue to acquire practices and build larger
and larger physician networks, there also is a steady stream of "leakage"—physicians who have concluded that hospital employment
simply isn't for them.

While I can't predict whether this trend will reach the level of
"disintegration" that hospitals and physicians reached in the late
1990s, the trend is irrefutably present. Clearly, many of these happy
marriages are showing signs of stress and aren't going to survive.
This *Physician's Guide to Returning to Private Practice* was written
to acknowledge this trend and provide physicians and their advisors
with a ready guide to the issues and pitfalls a decision to choose
independence will entail.

In my book, *Time to Sell? Guide to Selling a Physician Practice*,
which was originally published in 2008 and was revised in a third edition in 2016, I provide physicians with a pathway to selling their practices. *Time to Sell?* also recounts the pitfalls of such a huge decision.
As I originally predicted back in 2008, the sale of physician practices
to hospitals and health systems has continued relatively unabated.
Fueled further by the Affordable Care Act of 2010, this trend is now
showing some early signs of flaming out in some markets.

In early 2013, my company, which has been providing consulting
services in "the business of physician practice" to physicians and

hospitals since 1991, started to see the first inklings of what we call "disintegration." This disintegration is the opposite of the healthcare theme of *integration* that is as common now as it was when we started our company 25 years ago.

This emerging trend was wholly predictable. When I reflect on the changes between the first edition of *Time to Sell?* in 2008 through the second edition in 2011 and now the third edition in 2015, each publication included more red flags and warning signs. What began as a much more reasoned approach to hospital acquisition and employment of physicians morphed into higher valuations and unsustainable compensation structures.

These "front-end" mistakes predictably resulted in higher-than-expected losses for the hospital systems. Now the time has come to try to reduce those losses and, faced with that prospect, many physicians simply believe they can do better on their own. It isn't all driven by basic economics either—even physicians who recognize that their incomes may go down if they choose independence are choosing that route anyway because they want their autonomy back.

This guide arose out of my company's experiences in helping physicians navigate these tricky waters. In some cases we conducted feasibility studies on the issue for physician clients and recommended against taking this path back toward independence and they choose to do it anyway. There is a common refrain: "never underestimate man's desire for freedom." Some might use another refrain to physicians seeking to go back into private practice: "never underestimate man's stupidity." I'll let you decide which applies in your situation.

CHAPTER 1

Initial Considerations

Most of my colleagues who are employed by hospitals are
miserable.
ANONYMOUS PHYSICIAN

REESTABLISHING PRIVATE PRACTICE?

A re you crazy? That question may come from your spouse, your physician colleagues, or even your trusted CPA or practice consultant. Why, in this current healthcare environment, would you even consider going back into private practice?

The idea of returning to private practice manifests in many ways. For some, it appears almost like a dream, maybe even a bad one, and you wake up wondering if it was a nightmare or if you've lost your mind. For others it is more akin to a moment of clarity—you never imagined working for a hospital could be this bad. It can be a clear-cut economic decision. Or maybe economics don't matter, you just want your practice and your autonomy back.

Sometimes the hospital grass isn't greener. Sometimes even the money isn't worth it. If you've reached the stage where you are wishing for the "good old days" of private practice or if you are a younger physician and think you simply need to be in control of your own destiny, I understand, even if your spouse and your colleagues don't. The reality is, employment in a large organization is not for everyone.

Many of my healthcare consulting colleagues in competing firms (we're friendly competitors) and I have been fortunate enough to have long and successful careers as independent consultants. We often joke that we are "otherwise unemployable." We recognize this is an almost universal truth for us based on our personalities. This is also a universal truth for a subset of physicians. It's not for me to analyze what drives this truth for you, but if you are embarking down this road, you need to know yourself.

However you reached the point of seriously considering a return to private practice, know this: It isn't going to be easy or cheap and, as you will see, it isn't for everyone.

Questions, Questions, and More Questions

Where do you start? If you are a physician in a hospital employment relationship and are seriously considering establishing or reestablishing a private practice, you should begin by recognizing that this will not be your father's practice. The world has changed, and reestablishing what you had probably is not the way to go. Look at this as a fresh start. Look at it as an opportunity to create something totally new and different—as a way to avoid being a prisoner of your past experiences.

So, the first step is to carefully consider the vision of what you want your practice to be. That vision can be guided by questions such as these:

- Do I want to be in solo practice?
- If not, who will I practice with? Who will my partners and associates be?
- What about a small group?
- What about joining an existing independent group?
- Single-specialty or multispecialty?
- Are there others as miserable as me and will anyone want to do this together?
- Who will I share call with?
- Should I look at alternative practice models such as a concierge practice?

- Will the hospital compete with me?
- What are the terms of my contract with the hospital and can I get out of it?
- Do I have a noncompete?
- Will I be able to get payors to contract with me?
- Who will be my office manager and key staff?
- Where will I find key staff and what will they cost?
- What benefits will my staff want and what will that cost?
- How will I do billing and collections?
- What about electronic health records and other technology?
- How much will it cost to get started? Where will I get the money?
- What if the money doesn't come in?
- Can I get financing? Where? How? At what cost?
- What will my income be?
- Will I have to go without income for a while? How long?
- Where will my practice be located?
- Should I own my own building?
- What about furniture and equipment? What will I need? What will it cost? Where will I get it?
- Who will be my trusted advisors: attorney, CPA, and practice consultant?
- Will my patients follow me?

Answering these questions and the many others that come up will take some time, thought, and effort. Obviously not all of these questions will apply to everyone, and some of the answers may be obvious to you while others are more troublesome. Some questions may be unanswerable.

However, the important question to ask at this stage is this: *What did I like and dislike about private practice before, and what will I do differently this time?*

PERSPECTIVE—THE CYCLE OF PHYSICIAN EMPLOYMENT

Sometimes when we are in the middle of turmoil or facing important decisions, it's helpful to take a step back to gain some perspective. One key perspective is that hospital employment of physicians seems to be following a cycle that went full circle in the 1990s.

The short version is that beginning in the early 1990s, hospitals went on a huge acquisition binge, buying and employing physicians. The buying frenzy drove up acquisition prices and physician compensation to levels that were unsustainable. When the inevitable losses hit the bottom line, bond ratings and stock prices declined and CEOs were fired. Physician practices were unceremoniously divested in a similar binge fashion.

The long version of what I call the "Cycle of Physician Employment" is described in more detail in Appendix A. An understanding of this cycle provides two useful takeaways:
1. History that is repeating itself give us insight into the future, and
2. Those insights into the future allow us to predict what actions likely are coming and how and when we can use them to our advantage.

This Cycle of Physician Employment is unfolding differently in each market. Knowing and understanding where your hospital employer is in this cycle can be invaluable in both your decision-making and negotiating strategy if you are seriously considering a return to private practice.

WHY IT'S IMPORTANT

In general, the further a hospital is into this cycle, the more malleable (or even supportive) they may be to a physician seeking to leave employment and return to independent practice. The hospital's drive to dramatically reduce losses removes barriers to departure fairly quickly.

For example, in the late 1990s we saw hospital systems virtually giving the physicians back their practices. In some cases, hospitals paid physicians severance to terminate their contracts early and paid for consulting fees to support the physicians going back on their own—all in the interest of getting the losses off their books as soon as possible.

You can see, then, how important it might be to know where your hospital employer is in this cycle. If they have reached or are close to reaching the stage in the cycle where operating losses from physician employment are unsustainable, they may be willing to *pay* you to terminate your employment agreement early and fund some or all of the feasibility and other startup costs associated with you going back on your own.

Some hospitals will reject both of these tactics as illegal out of hand, but they aren't. Hospitals paying severance and feasibility costs to affect an early termination in order to reduce future operating losses is a common business survival strategy we've seen many times. It is defensible from both a financial and legal perspective so long as the amounts paid are less than what the future losses would have been. Both of these tactics are discussed further in Chapter 4.

Take a few minutes and review Appendix A to become more familiar with the details of the Cycle of Physician Employment. The checklist that follows Appendix A will aid you in assessing where your hospital is in this cycle.

ALTERNATIVE PRACTICE MODELS

Physicians disenchanted with hospital employment but unsure they want to reestablish and face the difficult realities of the typical Medicare and commercial insurance-based private practice model may want to consider alternative practice models. These models, such as concierge, retainer-based, and direct-pay practices, typically are suitable only for primary care physicians and have increasing appeal in many parts of the country.

In some ways, the Affordable Care Act hastened the development of these alternative practice models. The promise that healthcare reform would provide access to health insurance for an additional 25 million uninsured Americans turned out to be (mostly) true. Unfortunately for both providers and patients alike, the definition of "insurance" wasn't what many expected. A vast majority of this "new" health insurance coverage turned out to be high-deductible plans with correspondingly high co-insurance, providing insurance coverage for major health issues but not a plan that pays for most routine care.

Many physicians found that these high-deductible plans actually *decreased* cash flow while making it more difficult to monitor and collect patient balances. For example, many of these new plans limit or even eliminate coverage for office visits subject to the simple co-payment—a system most physician offices had become used to collecting and managing. Applying office visit charges to the patient's deductible leaves the physician's staff responsible not only for collecting 100% of the allowable charge directly from the patient, but also having to navigate and understand the dozens of varying plan terms and provisions.

In addition, in spite of promises that "you can keep your doctor," commercial insurers were allowed to develop "narrow networks" of providers. Many of these networks offered such low rates of reimbursement that many physicians simply opted not to join. Consequently, this system is driving both the patients and physicians to alternative models.

The affluent pre-Medicare-age baby boomer demographic is a prime target for these alternative practices. Consider the concierge practice, for example. For a typical monthly fee of $150 to $200, a patient gets same-day or next-day appointments that are much longer than the typical 15 minutes. They feel they have the attention of the physician who isn't rushing out to the next exam room. A typical concierge physician sees 8 to 10 patients per day and has a patient base of only about 600 patients compared to 2,500 to 3,000 in a typical primary care practice. The result is happier physicians and patients.

The math works, too. A typical primary care physician in private practice collects about $500,000 to $600,000 per year before overhead. A typical concierge physician with 600 patients paying $2,000 per year would collect $1.2 million—double.

Many concierge physicians are part of a concierge practice firm such as MDVIP, Paladina, Qliance, and MedLion. These firms can take as much as 33% of the revenue to provide administrative support, marketing, and other assistance in establishing and maintaining the concierge practice. That still leaves the physician with $800,000—a significant increase in revenue. In addition, it is likely that overhead will be reduced because many of the billing functions are reduced or eliminated as well.

These models not only allow the physician to spend more time with each patient and offer same- or next-day appointments, but the physician can get to know the patient and help with the patient's wellness, too. While critics lament the likelihood that concierge practices will hasten the shortage of primary care physicians, what did they expect when the healthcare system is allowed to continually devalue primary care physicians?

The biggest risk in establishing a concierge practice is in attracting the 600+ patients who are willing to pay the $2,000 or so per year. A careful assessment of the age and income demographics of the population in your service area and a sound marketing strategy are prerequisites to a successful concierge practice. There are also legal hurdles that need to be navigated in establishing concierge practices that can vary from state to state, so experienced legal counsel should be consulted before moving in this direction.

Several additional alternative models can be considered. For example, many commercial insurers are promoting telemedicine, which can supplement a physician's income during down time or provide a flow of patients with minimal overhead. Specialists can consider an on-call practice, in which they see consults or pre-/post-operative patients in a primary care office and maintain no physical office of their own. Micro-practices, in which physicians work out of one small room with little or no staff, and physicians who work from a fully equipped medical van and make house calls are some of the other alternative models we see in certain markets.

CHOOSING WHOM TO PRACTICE WITH

All physicians have a history, whether they have been in private practice or in a group practice. For those who were in a group, the history includes how the providers came to practice together. Group practice is like a marriage: Sometimes the choice of partners and associates wasn't well thought out or was based on compromises. Sometimes troubling personal characteristics don't show up until after the wedding. It's important to take some time and objectively consider previous experiences. What worked, what didn't, and what will you do differently this time around?

Sometimes choosing whom to practice with is an easy decision. Bonds often exist with colleagues from previous groups, and while the group may be employed by the hospital, all of the providers still practice in the same location and appear to the public as a group practice. This provides a logical answer to this question of whom to partner with. But sometimes it isn't quite that easy.

More commonly there has been turnover since the original sale of the practice. Older physicians may have retired or are slowing down. Younger physicians may have been added. These circumstances can present problems.

Physicians nearing retirement age may not be interested in investing time and risking capital in starting a practice that they will be involved with for a relatively short time. Conversely, younger physicians are often risk-averse when it comes to business. Oftentimes they have not been in private practice and lack both understanding of and interest in what is involved.

Both the older and younger physicians may overtly or covertly seek to remain employees of the hospital which, depending on your specialty and the specifics of the situation (number of physicians involved, competing practices, call coverage issues, etc.), can make returning to private practice difficult and, in some cases, virtually impossible.

Hospitals are pretty adept at ferreting out these situations fairly quickly, and you can expect them to use them to their advantage as the negotiations unfold. That said, it is also important to recognize the motivation of the hospital. Again, depending on your specialty, group size, competition in your specialty, and many other factors, it could be that the hospital prefers you stay together as a group.

It's equally important to recognize that in forming a new group practice, you are no longer bound to the legacy organization structure of the group you originally sold to the hospital. That group is gone and it is likely that the legal entity that it operated under is gone, too. And even if that entity still is in legal existence, you are not required to use it. When starting a new group, you can begin with a blank page, and that means you can violate some of the old-standing "rules" of group practice that date back to the 1960s, when practices first started to organize as corporations.

For example, everyone does not have to be an owner or partner. You can explore structures that allow younger physicians to be employees into perpetuity, if that better suits your situation. Older physicians approaching retirement or already in slow-down mode likewise can be employees. Obviously the trick with these models is rewarding those who are willing to take the business risk while still meeting the compensation expectations of those who are not.

When starting a new group, meeting the needs of older physicians nearing retirement is generally much easier. For example, whatever arrangement is put in place has a limited term that can be established in advance based on a future retirement date.

Younger physicians can be more of a challenge and the pitfalls can be huge. Combining risk-averseness on the business side with salary expectations that may not reflect the underlying economic reality of private practice can lead to irreconcilable differences. While it may be possible to work through the lack of ownership and financial risk, compensation expectations need to follow, and generally they don't.

Part of the problem is that salaries paid by the hospitals don't reflect economic reality. In private practice, physician compensation is generally what is left after paying overhead, which is a true reflection of the economic earnings of that physician. The survey data that many employed physicians have come to rely on as indicative of what they are worth in terms of salary is distorted. As more physicians have become employees of hospitals, survey responses are increasingly dominated with physicians employed by hospital systems. Hospitals generate significant losses on employed physicians and the salaries reported in the surveys are artificially subsidized. The magnitude of these subsidies is included in Appendix A.

Here again, the specifics of your situation come into play. Many physicians seeking to leave hospital employment do so in the face of compensation "restructuring"—a code word for reduction in compensation. If that is the case, the reality of those cuts affects everyone, and this may help lower the compensation expectations of younger physicians.

However, younger physicians are more mobile, and high levels of school debt and other financial pressures tend to make it easier for them to search for a higher guaranteed salary, absent the potential financial risk of private practice, by relocating to a different part of the country. Practice autonomy and cultural considerations are inclined to be more important to the older physicians than compensation. The converse is true for younger physicians.

As you work through these issues and discussions, don't ignore the most important facet: cultural fit of your potential colleagues. The common bond that can be formed among a group of physicians who decide to separate from hospital employment can sometimes be akin to a shotgun wedding. This common desire to be out from under the hospital, for whatever reason, can mask the need for a critical examination of the cultural fit of the physicians involved.

Ask yourself whether this group of individuals is the group you would choose to go into practice with if you had total freedom of choice. Listen carefully in your discussions with them, consider their business acumen and business behavior, and take an objective look at the likely cultural fit. Imagine yourself in partner meetings or board meetings with these individuals and consider their willingness and ability to engage in the complex decision making and related financial risk that may follow some of those decisions.

Don't ignore clinical considerations either. The overarching question above bears repeating: Is this the group of individuals I would choose to go into practice with if I had total freedom of choice?

In the 1990s, when my company was merging as many as 15 or 20 small independent groups into large single-specialty and multispecialty group practices, one of my former partners had an effective—and disarming—comment for those who didn't seem to fit into the culture the new group was trying to create. He'd simply say, "Doctor, this may not be for you," and leave it at that.

Making concessions to get 100% consensus or to meet the lowest common denominator is not in your best interest nor the best interest of the group you are trying to create. It is better to leave some people behind than to compromise principles that risk the long-term success of the business.

INITIAL STEPS

One of the biggest mistakes in returning to private practice is reaching the decision hastily and taking insufficient time to develop a plan that identifies and takes into account past lessons. Returning to private practice properly requires an investment of both time and money. Trying to go down this road without an objective and trusted advisor to work with you through the steps in a deliberate manner is the biggest mistake you can make.

This might mean going along and getting along in your current, and perhaps untenable, situation for longer than you'd prefer. Even if you are independently wealthy and can afford to throw money at a snap, emotional decision to reestablish private practice out of anger (or even distain) for your hospital employer, moving too quickly will likely sow the seeds for difficulties that could have been avoided.

Figure 1 illustrates the major steps you will need to go through as you consider leaving hospital employment and reestablishing yourself in private practice.

These steps include:

1. *Initial considerations.* An examination of your motivations, who you will practice with, how to get started, and how long it might take.
2. *Legal considerations.* An examination of the critical legal issues surrounding a potential separation, including whether the hospital will let you go, restrictive covenants, etc.
3. *Feasibility and financing.* An objective (and crucial) examination of the financial feasibility of reestablishing private practice, including estimates of startup costs and examination of financing options and availability.

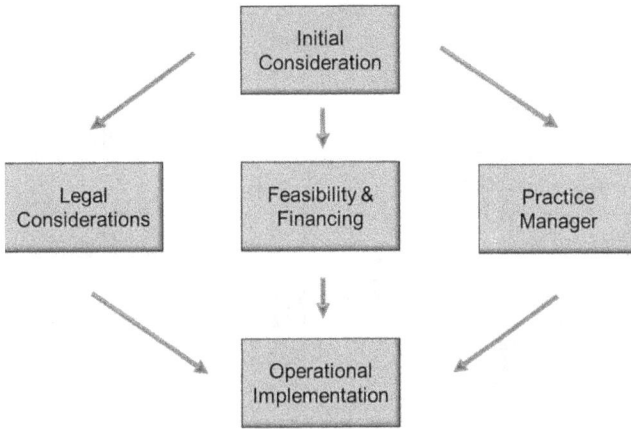

FIGURE 1. Major considerations when reestablishing private practice.

4. *Management.* Assuming the decision is made to proceed, the critical steps of identifying and hiring a practice manager and other key staff who will complete, in conjunction with you other advisors, the operational implementation of the new group.

These steps are examined in detail in the following chapters and will address three key initial questions:

- Is the separation possible legally?
- Does it make sense financially?
- Will the hospital be supportive or resist?

You may have already answered some of these questions, but as you will see, verbal discussions don't always translate into legal agreements.

In addition, you should consider whether all participants are on the same page with respect to what is driving the group formation and can they reach a fundamental understanding and consensus on the basic financial, cash flow, and strategy that form the basis for the group's business plan? Do they understand what the group formation will mean for and require of the individual physician participants?

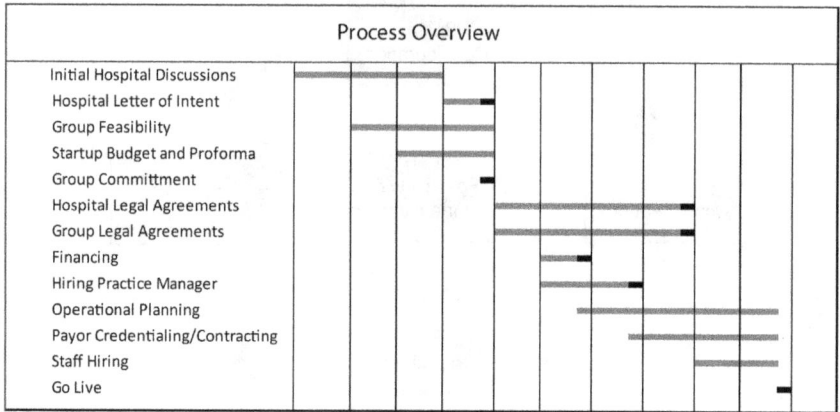

FIGURE 2. Process of separating from hospital and establishing private practice.

The first three steps will require some initial level of financial investment by interested physicians, although in some situations, as discussed above, the hospital may be willing to fund the initial feasibility. However, the willingness of potential participants to write a personal check to get started will provide insight into who is really serious. These steps will ultimately lead to a go/no-go decision on whether to move forward.

UNFOLDING THE PROCESS

Before we address the details of moving forward, let's step back and look at a brief overview of how the entire process of separating from a hospital and reestablishing private practice unfolds.

Figure 2 provides an overview of the typical process; steps are described briefly below and explored in greater detail in the following chapters.

The typical process is as follows:

1. The initial discussions with the hospital will answer the question of whether a separation is possible. If it is, proceed with the feasibility phase, which will lead to a go/no-go decision. The end result

of these two initiatives typically is a letter of intent (LOI) with the hospital and a commitment or LOI among the physicians to proceed with forming the group.

2. The next steps from a legal standpoint are twofold: proceed with formalizing the separation agreement with the hospital and proceed with forming the group's legal entity and formalizing the group's agreements between the physicians.

3. While these legal agreements are being drafted and negotiated, the group arranges financing, hires a practice manager, and proceeds with operational planning, which includes provider number transfers, payor contracting, credentialing, staffing, and all the other tasks necessary to ready the group for a future go-live date on which the physicians commence practicing as an independent group.

HOW LONG WILL IT TAKE?

When you sold your practice and became an employee of the hospital, any cash flow issues arising out of payor contracting and credentialing and other billing issues likely didn't impact you financially. The opposite is true this time around. While there is always a drive to get the deal done, especially after the decision to divorce has been made, caution is in order.

The biggest financial risk you have here concerns the revenue cycle: provider number transfers, payor contracting, credentialing, and the systems that ensure claims are filed and that accounts receivable are collected on a timely basis.

Once the decision has been made to separate, the hospital likely will want you gone as soon as possible. They may be experiencing significant financial losses and want those losses off the books sooner rather than later. This puts their financial interests directly at odds with your need to have sufficient time to ensure you are fully prepared and everything is in place.

In addition, in my experience, the hospital's desire for your quick departure usually is not matched by any kind of expediency from their legal counsel. Most large hospital systems use in-house counsel, and in-house counsel often lacks decision-making ability. The separation agreements generally require a lot of negotiation and are not typically a standard agreement their counsel has a lot of experience in drafting. These factors conspire to prolong the process.

When estimating how long it will take to reestablish private practice, I suggest you start with a minimum of six months after you have made the decision to move forward upon completion of the feasibility study; nine months is more realistic. You cannot put your financial future at risk to meet someone else's artificial timetable. You should also recognize, however, that the longer the process draws out, the higher your startup costs become, because legal consulting and other pre-operational expenses continue until you reach the go-live date and start to generate charges that ultimately lead to cash flow.

CHAPTER 2

Legal Considerations

Don't read the chapter title and turn the page.
THE AUTHOR

This chapter addresses the first critical steps you should take after deciding to consider returning to private practice.

Regardless of the discussions you may have had with the hospital or what your peers and colleagues have told you in the doctor's lounge, you need to know and understand exactly what your contract with the hospital says—you need to know your legal status. Perhaps the hospital has already told you verbally you are free to leave. Perhaps friends or colleagues have already left and told you how the separation was structured. It doesn't matter. What do *your* agreements stipulate?

Regardless of what has been said to or promised to or done for others, make no mistake about it, there will be negotiations. Before entering into any negotiation, you need to know where the power lies. By that I mean, what does the hospital have control over in the existing agreements that you need or want them to waive or change?

In the typical sale of a practice to a hospital, there are two main contractual agreements: the physician employment agreement and the asset purchase agreement. What do they say, if anything, about what happens in the case of termination?

EMPLOYMENT AGREEMENT

The employment agreement is usually the most important because it likely includes some kind of restrictive covenant or noncompete language that may affect your options. Even if the hospital has verbally agreed to waive these provisions, when the hospital attorneys become involved, strings will probably be attached. Understanding what is required by the contract language has to be your starting point.

Begin by summarizing, in writing, your understanding of the existing employment agreement. Outline any discussions you have had with the hospital and generate a list of questions you have. Then engage experienced legal counsel to review the agreement, confirm or deny your understanding, and answer your questions. The goal is to come away with an understanding of exactly where you stand and a strategy for having your attorney *negotiate on your behalf* to get you what you want and need to affect the separation.

The best and most efficient way to approach this separation is through a letter of intent (LOI). While LOIs generally are not binding, they are an invaluable way to get all the issues on the table and to move both parties toward an efficient separation.

Physician employment contracts can vary widely. What does your contract say with respect to a noncompete, returning to private practice, terminating employment with the hospital? Many noncompetes today shy away from forcing physicians to leave a community in the event of termination because in many areas, it is difficult to recruit replacement physicians. Often the only restriction is on selling or affiliating with a competitor of your current hospital employer, and that leaves open the option of returning to private practice.

Often these types of noncompetes limit the return to private practice to the structure of the practice before it was sold. But what if you aren't selling to or joining a competing hospital and aren't really interested in reestablishing private practice with the physicians you were in practice with? What if some of them have retired and their replacements or even some of your former partners aren't interested in leaving hospital employment? What if there is another single-specialty or multispecialty group you'd like to join? Write down your thoughts, concerns, and answers to these types of questions and discuss them with your attorney, who might offer a different perspective.

Even if there is a full restrictive covenant or noncompete clause that prohibits you from practicing within so many miles of the hospital or one of its facilities, it may not apply, depending on the provision the contract will be terminated under. Review your employment agreement and look for and understand any termination provisions. The manner in which the agreement will be terminated often affects how the noncompete applies.

Most employment agreements include more than one termination provision. Typical provisions include a termination with cause provision, a termination without cause provision, and sometimes a termination upon expiration or nonrenewal of the contract. Your focus should be on which of these provisions, if any, might apply in your situation. For example, if the contract is terminated for breach by the hospital or terminated by either party without cause (if the contract provides for such termination), or if the contract expires without renewal, the noncompete may be waived.

In cases where the hospital has verbally agreed to waive the restrictive covenant, your attorney will still need to read and understand the contract language to assure the LOI and the formal contracts documenting the agreed-upon separation terms reflect these verbal agreements.

When faced with a strong restrictive covenant and a hospital that opposes a physician's desire to leave, physicians who are angry and dissatisfied with their current employment relationship often threaten lawsuits to overturn noncompete clauses. The enforceability of noncompete clauses and restrictive covenants varies widely by state, and this is another area in which you will want experienced legal counsel.

Threatening or pursuing lawsuits, especially in the early stages, generally is not a winning strategy for two reasons. First, the noncompete likely was originally drafted by experienced attorneys hired by the hospital and they believe there is a high probability it will be upheld. Second, the hospital probably doesn't want you to leave the community anyway, regardless what the contract states.

If they have a reasonable expectation of your continued support, a negotiated separation is often more plausible than you might think, even in situations where there is initial resistance to you leaving.

Looking beyond the legal language to the hospital's motivation is another key consideration. Regardless what the contracts say, anything is negotiable if two parties are motivated and the agreement is legal. In many cases, hospitals are more than willing, for any number of reasons, to divest themselves of unhappy physicians. Unhappy doctors who are perceived as not fitting in with the majority of the employed physicians or who are not viewed as "team players" don't fit their desire for a manageable and largely compliant physician network.

Don't let your ego be damaged if this is how you are perceived—use it to your advantage. A well-known adage in hospital circles is that managing physicians is like herding cats. So what if you are the tomcat on the prowl, the outlier? Use the fact that they may be glad to be rid of you to your advantage, because that's what you want also. As noted above, hospitals are often motivated by getting the losses off their books and a divestiture is the quickest way to do so.

COMPENSATION CONSIDERATIONS

Termination of the employment agreement also could give rise to compensation issues, depending on your current compensation structure. Unless you are compensated on a straight salary, compensation is generally determined by a formal compensation plan document, which is usually an attachment to the employment agreement. These compensation plans tend to be complex and can be vague or subject to interpretation about what happens in the event of termination.

Many compensation plans provide for bonuses, incentive payments, or other compensation that is payable on a quarterly or annual basis.

Often these plans include provisions that limit the payment bonuses or other incentives to physicians who are employed at the time such payment is actually made.

Physicians whose compensation is all or partially based on net revenue, as opposed to actual cash collections, should ensure the net revenue estimates made by the hospital accurately reflect actual collection experience. The differences between the cash basis method of recognizing revenue most physicians in private practice use versus the accrual basis method hospitals use is something you may need your CPA or practice consultant to look at. This issue and the calculations and analysis can be complex and likely will require several years' worth of gross charge and actual collection data for a complete analysis.

We recently worked with a group that was leaving hospital employment and found the hospital had underestimated net revenue over the five-year period preceding the separation by several hundred thousand dollars, so don't ignore this analysis if a component of your compensation is net revenue.

As stated above, everything is negotiable in the right situation. Contract provisions may seem to put you at a disadvantage, but in the right situation, even these provisions can be rectified. If they can't, it may be necessary to delay or time your departure to ensure you receive any payments you believe you have earned and are entitled to. For example, if an annual bonus is only payable if you are still employed at the time, consider delaying your departure.

ASSET PURCHASE AGREEMENT

The asset purchase agreement you signed as part of the original sale should also be reviewed. Under the terms of this agreement, you sold the hospital-specified assets of the practice for a specified price with specified terms.

Which assets were included? Did the sale include intangible assets such as the practice's name, phone number, and patient records, even if a separate value was assigned to these items? Are there any provisions in the asset purchase agreement that apply in the case of termination? Some asset purchase agreements, especially where intangible assets were sold, include specific provisions that apply in the event of termination. Such provisions may include a requirement that certain tangible and intangible assets be repurchased at a specified price or at current fair market value. The agreement may even specify how fair market value will be determined. Examples of these assets might include furniture and equipment, medical records, trained workforce in place, and even real estate.

Reviewing the asset purchase agreement for such provisions is another important and necessary step in understanding where you stand legally. It should be noted again that regardless what the agreements say, motivated parties can negotiate or renegotiate any agreement as long as it is legal. For example, while the purchase prices of your furniture and equipment may be negotiable, the hospital can't legally sell it back to you for less than its current fair market value. However, assuming most of the furniture and equipment consists of the same items you sold to the hospital several years ago, the odds are that the value will be less than what it was at that time.

MEDICAL RECORDS AND PATIENT DEMOGRAPHIC DATA

One final and important consideration in the initial separation discussions is ensuring your access to the demographic data and medical records of your patients. The hospital should be willing to provide these data free of charge; otherwise, they would have the custodial responsibility to maintain the records for the prescribed statutory timeframe and comply with record requests from patients. Failure or resistance to providing these data would be foolhardy on the hospital's part because, presuming your patients will follow you, they could simply require the hospital to provide you copies of their records anyway.

Complexities do arise when the data are in electronic form and HIPPA requirements need to be considered as well. Electronic interfaces may be needed to transfer some or all of the data between the hospital's system and yours if you are converting to a different system, and you should expect to pay for that interface. Absent a previous agreement requiring you to repurchase the medical records, this information should be provided by the hospital for no charge beyond the cost of the required interface.

LEGAL TAKEAWAYS

Ideally, you want to create a situation in which both parties agree that a separation is the best course of action. Once you have accomplished that objective, working through any legal obstacles presented in the existing contacts becomes much easier.

However, if the hospital resists the separation or is unreasonable in its demands, *hire an experienced healthcare transaction attorney who has been through this drill before.* Investing in someone with extensive experience will put the hospital on notice that you are serious, and sometimes that in itself will bring a more civil discourse to the negotiations table.

CHAPTER 3

Feasibility

If the data doesn't support the desired conclusion, the data must be changed.

ANONYMOUS

After you have established a pathway through any legal issues with the hospital and tentatively identified physician participants, you need to assess the financial feasibility of the proposed venture.

The purpose of this feasibility assessment is to assure that all participants are on the same page with respect to what is driving the group formation and to reach a general understanding and consensus on the basic financial, cash flow, and strategy that form the foundation for the group's business plan. This includes consensus around what the group formation will mean to and require of the individual physician participants. Engaging an experienced consultant to take you through this process is critical.

The "art" of an effective feasibility process is to keep the focus on the key fundamental questions and decisions, and avoid being bogged down in operational and other decisions that can be deferred until later—these decisions only serve as a distraction at this point. For example, decisions about which bank, insurance agent, attorney, CPA, retirement plan, or billing/EHR software you are going to use are largely irrelevant at this stage of the process. The focus should be on vision and strategy, startup and operating costs, how you will make decisions, and cash flow/physician income projections. Set the detail issues aside until after you've made the decision to proceed.

This feasibility process should include the following steps:

1. Establish a common purpose and vision about what is driving the group's formation and ensure all physician participants are on the same page.

2. Examine and agree on the organization and governance structure of the group—how the new group will make decisions, whether a separate governing board will run the group, the size and composition of that board, and what decisions will require majority or supermajority votes. The group governance worksheet included at the end of this chapter outlines the types of issues that should be considered.

3. Outline the basic legal and economic relationships that will be developed among the participating members, such as ownership, employment, part-time physicians, buy-in and buy-out, etc. This outline should include an examination and discussion of some of the issues discussed earlier, such as varying perspectives between older and younger physicians.

4. Develop a detailed financial projection of startup costs, revenue, overhead expense, cash flow, physician compensation, and capital (borrowing) requirements that allows each participant to assess the financial impact the group will have on them personally. Should the group decide to move forward, these financial projections will support the group's efforts to secure financing. The financial analysis and projections should include the following components:
   - Projected startup and development costs;
   - Projected income statements for two years; and
   - Monthly cash flow projections for the first 24 months.

Let's look at each of these components in more detail.

PROJECTED STARTUP AND DEVELOPMENT COSTS

Startup and development costs include pre-operational "soft costs" necessary to get the group off the ground. These costs typically include legal, consulting, accounting, and pre-operational staffing costs such as your practice manager, who will need to be hired and on board several months before your go-live date.

As noted above and discussed in more detail below, it may be possible to get the hospital to agree to fund part or all of the cost of the feasibility study, especially if the hospital is motived to reduce its operating losses on employed physicians.

Other startup and development costs include capital expenditures to purchase furniture and equipment from the hospital or other sources, any space renovations or leasehold improvements for your office, and hardware and software costs for your practice management (billing) and electronic health records system.

In addition to pre-operational soft costs and capital expenditures, you will also need working capital. Working capital essentially means a funding source to cover operating overhead of the group such as staff salaries and benefits, rent, clinical and other operating expenses during the time it takes for your accounts receivable to ramp-up and be collected. This ramp-up is discussed in more detail below.

A startup capital worksheet is included at the end of this chapter to help you identify and estimate these costs. Potential financing sources are discussed in detail in Chapter 4.

PROJECTED INCOME STATEMENTS FOR TWO YEARS

The projected income statements serve two goals: (1) to allow each participant to assess the financial impact the group will have on them personally, and (2) to support the group's efforts to secure financing

The most accurate way to approach this is to start with your historical income statements under hospital employment and then overlay anticipated changes in your revenue and overhead in an independent group setting. Adjust or "roll-forward" each line item based on projected changes in revenue and overhead cost. Estimates are made and updated throughout the pre-operational process as decisions are made and cost estimates firmed up.

Sometimes the hospital's income statements will lack an adequately detailed expense breakdown. Other times the income statements may include physicians in other specialties or locations who will not be part of your new group. But starting with a base historical income statement and conducting a roll-forward is the best way to manage the development of these projections. In most cases, the hospital should be willing to provide this detailed information and an experienced practice consultant will know what questions to ask and how to develop accurate projections.

The biggest and most critical adjustment will be converting the hospital's accrual basis net revenue to a cash basis and then overlaying the impact of the "ramp-up" of accounts receivable.

Your new group will start with zero in accounts receivable and the gross charges you initially generate will take time to be collected. This is commonly known as the (accounts receivable) ramp-up period because during this time, your accounts receivable will be building up. Accounts receivable and monthly collections will typically stabilize after three to four months at a normal level. During these initial months, your cash collections will be less than what they will ultimately be on a typical monthly basis.

The resulting impact on cash flow will need to be funded through the various financing mechanisms discussed in Chapter 4, typically through a working capital line of credit from your bank, secured by your accounts receivable. It is important to recognize that this cash flow is not lost, it is simply deferred. Accounts receivable represent a significant asset of the practice and serve as ready collateral for this working capital line of credit (see Chapter 4).

Other typical overhead adjustments that need to be made in this roll-forward include the following:

1. Staff salaries and benefits need to be adjusted to reflect the staffing levels, salary rates, and benefits you will offer your employees as an independent group.
2. Clinical expenses need to be adjusted to reflect the services you will provide through your office (medical supplies, lab, x-ray, drugs and injectables, etc.) based on vendor contracts you negotiate.
3. Building and occupancy costs need to be adjusted to reflect the rent and occupancy costs of the group on a standalone basis. If the group owns its office space, rent should be adjusted to reflect the rent you will charge yourselves.
4. Furniture and equipment costs need to be adjusted to reflect any equipment leases you assume from the hospital or enter into on your own. Costs for maintenance and maintenance contracts need to be estimated as well.
5. Administrative expenses should reflect your decisions about promoting and marketing the practice and about information technology (IT) such as software licensing costs and IT support. Transcription costs, interest on borrowing, outside professional fees, and other administrative cost also should be considered.
6. Professional liability and general liability insurance costs should be adjusted as premium quotes are obtained.
7. Finally, overhead and other cost allocations from the hospital to your income statement need to be eliminated.

These adjustments are estimated during the initial feasibility. If the decision is made to move forward with the group, as noted above, these estimates are updated throughout the pre-operational process as decisions are made and cost estimates firmed up. The income statement worksheet at the end of this chapter illustrates the suggested layout and approach and includes samples of the typical roll-forward adjustments that should be considered.

The projected income statements also should include a projection of future incomes of the individual physician owners and form the basis for monthly cash flow projections, including estimates of any working capital borrowing needs, account receivable ramp-up, and debt service requirements.

MONTHLY CASH FLOW PROJECTION FOR TWO YEARS

Think of the monthly cash flow projection as a deeper and more granular look at the projected income statements discussed above. The annual projections are broken down to a monthly basis in order to give you a more specific projection of your expected collections, overhead, and working capital borrowing needs. It is not as simple as taking the projected annual income statements and dividing them by 12, because most of the working capital borrowing will need to occur during your first few months of operations due to the accounts receivable ramp-up.

Other questions to consider: What is your borrowing capacity? Do your borrowing needs exceed your borrowing capacity or will you have unused capacity (a cushion)? Which month has the highest borrowing? How long will it take to pay off your line of credit? What impact do things like physician salary deferrals (sweat equity), vendor terms, payroll dates, and myriad other decisions have on this equation?

FEASIBILITY SUMMARY

Upon completion, the feasibility process will provide a blueprint for the formation of the group and sufficient information to allow individual physicians to decide whether to pursue separation from the hospital.

Should the feasibility study result in a decision by a sufficient number of physicians to go forward as a group, those physicians should enter into a more formal letter of intent to join the new group and to move ahead toward funding the startup costs and the hiring of legal counsel to negotiate with the hospital and draft the legal agreements for the group, as well as other advisors, such as consultants and CPAs, necessary to begin operational planning.

While the group formation typically is not legally binding until these formal contracts have been drafted and executed, the nature of the financial commitments and decisions that must be planned and implemented after this point make it difficult for physicians to drop out. Generally, a commitment at this stage should be viewed as a commitment to join the new group.

GROUP GOVERNANCE WORKSHEET

Note: The purpose of the worksheet is to facilitate initial discussion and planning on group governance issues. Items in this worksheet are subject to specific legal language to be subsequently developed by legal counsel and may be subject to specific legal issues in various jurisdictions. This worksheet should not be utilized without the advice of legal counsel.

Shareholders

1. A quorum of the shareholders (shareholder = partner) will be:
   - ❏ A majority of shareholders in attendance
   - ❏ A majority of shareholders in the group
   - ❏ A majority of shareholders in attendance plus written proxies held
   - ❏ Other
2. Supermajority votes of the shareholders will be % of:
   - ❏ Total shareholders in the group
   - ❏ Shareholders in attendance
   - ❏ Shareholders in attendance plus written proxies held
   - ❏ Other
3. Shareholder meetings will be held:
   - ❏ Monthly
   - ❏ Quarterly
   - ❏ Annually
   - ❏ Other
   - ❏ Shareholder decisions can be made without a meeting by written vote

Board

4. The Board will consist of:
   - ❏ All shareholders
   - ❏ _____ shareholders
   - ❏ _____ shareholders from each site

❑ Non-shareholder physicians at the discretion of the shareholders

5. Board nominations will be from:
   ❑ A nominating committee of _____ elected by the shareholders
   ❑ At-large nominations from the floor
   ❑ Other _____

6. Board terms
   ❑ There will be an initial Board that will serve a term of _____ years
   ❑ Board terms will be staggered __ 1 year, __ 2 years, __ 3 years
   ❑ There will be no term limits
   ❑ Board members will be limited to no more than _____ consecutive terms
   ❑ Other

7. Board action requires:
   ❑ A majority of Board members in attendance
   ❑ A majority of Board members in attendance plus written proxies held
   ❑ Other

8. Board compensation will be:
   ❑ None
   ❑ Set by Board
   ❑ Set by Board and ratified by shareholders

9. ❑ Board Committees will be set by the Board
   ❑ Board Committees will be:
      – Finance
      – Operations
      – Compensation
      – Managed care contracting
      – Other _____
      – Other _____
      – Other _____
   ❑ Board Committees may include:
      – Shareholders only
      – Non-shareholders

10. Board and shareholder powers will be divided as follows: (Powers not reserved to the shareholders revert to the Board, subject to state law review.)

		Shareholder Majority	Shareholder Super-Majority	Board
a.	Hire a mid-level provider			
b.	Hire a physician provider			
c.	Admit a new shareholder			
d.	Operating budget approval			
e.	Capital budget approval			
f.	Change in shareholders' compensation plan			
g.	Borrow funds in excess of $ _____			
h.	Borrow funds in excess of $ _____ (requiring personal guarantees)			
i.	Borrow funds in excess of group line of credit (not requiring personal guarantees)			
j.	Make a commitment (lease, etc.) in excess of $_____ over the life of the lease			
k.	Enter into practice mergers			
l.	Enter into joint ventures			
m.	Enter into management agreements			
n.	Sell off all or part of the group			
o.	Amend the group's legal agreements			
p.	Terminate a shareholder physician with cause			
q.	Terminate a shareholder physician without cause			
r.				
s.				
t.				
u.				
v.				
w.				
x.				
y.				
z.				

STARTUP CAPITAL WORKSHEET

	Pre-Operational		Working
	Low	High	Capital
USES OF FUNDS			
Capital Expenditures			
Purchase Existing Furniture and Equipment			
Purchase New Furniture and Equipment			
Practice Management/EHR/Other Software			
Space Renovations/Leasehold Improvements			
Pre-Operational			
Consulting Feasibility and Operational Planning			
Legal Counsel—Hospital Negotiations			
Legal Counsel—Local-Group Agreements			
Accounting			
Practice Manager Salary & Benefits			
Other/Contingency			
Working Capital			
Ramp-up of Accounts Receivable			
Clinical Supply, Drugs And Injectable Inventory			
Total Uses of Funds			
SOURCES OF FUNDS			
Owners' Equity Investment			
Owners' Salary Deferral (Sweat Equity)			
Hospital Start-Up Support			
Hospital Equipment Lease			
Hospital Equipment Financing			
Assumption of Hospital PTO and/or Severance			
Bank Term Loan			

	Pre-Operational		Working
	Low	High	Capital
Bank Line of Credit			
Billing Company			
EHR Vendor Lease or PAYG Structure			
Vendor Terms on Clinic Supplies			
Other			
Total Sources of Funds			

INCOME STATEMENT WORKSHEET

	Historical Income Statement	Independent Group Adjustments	Projected Independent Group Year One
Revenue			
Medical Revenue		(1)	
Operating Cost **Salaries & Benefits, Non-Providers**			
Salaries		(2)	
Employee Benefits		(2)	
Clinical Expenses			
Medical Supplies		(3)	
Lab Expenses		(3)	
X-ray Expenses		(3)	
Drugs & Injectables		(3)	
Other Clinical Expenses		(3)	
Building & Occupancy			
Rent		(4)	
Building Maintenance & Repairs		(4)	
Utilities		(4)	
Other Building & Occupancy		(4)	
Furniture/Equipment			
Equipment Rental		(5)	
Equipment Maintenance & Repairs		(5)	
Debt Service		(6)	

(Continued on next page)

	Historical Income Statement	Independent Group Adjustments	Projected Independent Group Year One
Administrative Expenses			
Promotion & Marketing		(7)	
Telephone/Internet/Answering		(7)	
Service Transcription		(7)	
Outside Professional Fees		(7)	
Administrative Supplies & Services		(7)	
Other Administrative Expenses		(7)	
Billing Fees		(8)	
Software Licensing & Maintenance Fees		(9)	
Information Technology (IT Support)		(10)	
Hospital Allocations		(11)	
Interest Expense		(12)	
Insurance			
Insurance, Other		(7)	
Insurance, Professional Liability		(7)	
Total Operating Cost			
Available for Physician Compensation & Benefits			

INCOME STATEMENT ADJUSTMENTS WORKSHEET

Adjustment Number	Description	Initial Estimate	Updated Estimate	Final Estimate
(1)	Revenue adjustments			
	Accrual basis to cash collections			
	Accounts receivable ramp-up			
	Changes in service mix			
	Changes in provider base			
(2)	Staff salary and benefit costs			
	Number of full-time equivalent (FTE) staff			
	New hires, including practice manager			
	Terminations			
	Salary and hourly rate adjustments			
	Benefit package cost			
(3)	Clinical expenses based on vendor negotiations			
(4)	Building and occupancy costs based on space lease terms			
(5)	Furniture and equipment costs			
(6)	Equipment leases			
(6)	Equipment maintenance and maintenance agreements			
(7)	Debt service on equipment acquisition loan			
(8)	Billing fees to reflect terms of negotiated agreement			
(9)	Software licensing and maintenance fees based on applicable negotiated agreements			
(10)	Information technology (IT support) based on service agreement			
(11)	Eliminate any hospital allocation of overhead and support costs			
(12)	Interest expense on working capital line of credit based on cash flow projections			
(13)	Adjusted insurance based on current quotes			
(14)	Adjusted professional liability insurance based on current quotes			

CHAPTER 4

Financing

*If you would know the value of money, go and try to
borrow some.*
BENJAMIN FRANKLIN

SENIOR DEBT

In the current financial environment, bank debt is readily available in most parts of the country for established physicians who want to reestablish private practices on their own. Interest rates remain low, which makes bank debt financing, also called senior debt financing, the most viable option for most physicians.

The primary financing needs of a group are:

1. Funding startup "soft costs"—the initial consulting, legal, and accounting fees required to get the group off the ground. Soft costs also likely will need to fund salary and benefit costs for a group office manager or administrator who must be hired several months in advance of the group's separation or "go-live" date as well.

2. Equipment financing to acquire the furniture and equipment necessary to operate the practice.

3. Working capital to fund operating expenses and physician salaries during the accounts receivable ramp-up period—the initial three to six months of operations.

The startup capital worksheet at the end of Chapter 3 should help you summarize capital requirements and potential financing sources.

Banks generally will offer three basic types of financing:

1. A term loan for initial startup and soft costs. This loan will often be rolled into an installment loan for the furniture and equipment purchases when the group reaches that point.
2. An installment loan for furniture and equipment purchases.
3. A line of credit for working capital secured by your accounts receivable.

Although bank debt is readily available in most parts of the country, banks may view the practice as a startup business regardless of the number of years the participating physicians have been in practice. A startup business usually means the bank will undertake a higher level of due diligence and the financing likely will require some level of personal guarantees from the physicians.

Personal guarantees means that in the event of default by the group, the bank has the right to pursue repayment from the personal assets of the individual physicians (the "guarantors") should the collateral provided by the group be insufficient to satisfy the obligation.

This is another area where your feasibility efforts will pay off. Most banks love to gain physician clients and to loan money to physicians, but they will want to see income and cash flow projections supporting the group's ability to repay its borrowing. Being able to provide the professionally prepared and detailed financial projections developed during your feasibility phase will support your efforts to secure financing and often mitigate the level of personal guarantees.

Personal guarantees come in three basic forms:

- *Joint liability.* The bank has the right to pursue any or all of the guarantors for the full amount of the debt.
- *Several liability.* This is also known as proportionate liability, meaning the bank has the right to pursue each guarantor only for the amount of his or her "share" of the liability. For example, if five physicians borrowed $100,000 with several liability through personal guarantees, the bank could pursue each guarantor for their pro rata share of the obligation, which in this example is $20,000.

Several liability is often set at a higher percentage of a pro rata share, and this percentage is often negotiable. For example, banks that offer several liability may ask each guarantor be liable for 125% of a pro rata share, so instead of the $20,000 in the above example, each physician would be liable for $25,000 (125% times $20,000).

- *Joint and several liability.* This combines the two such that if the bank pursues and receives payment from one guarantor, that guarantor is free to pursue action against the other guarantors for their respective shares of the liability.

Whenever possible, avoid banks that require joint or joint and several liability guarantees because personal guarantees of this nature can be a source of a major divide when starting a new group. Younger physicians are unlikely to have as much net worth as the older physicians, and when joint or joint and several personal guarantees are required, this puts the older physicians at higher risk, which they generally are not willing to take.

At the same time, younger physicians with limited net worth and risk-averseness tend to view any form of personal guarantee with major concern. They are early in their careers and may have substantial school debt remaining. Taking on even a share of the risk through a several liability guarantee can be a major burden.

When confronting these issues in your discussions, it is important to recognize that even in the worst case, the personal guarantees come into play only after the assets the practice put up as collateral have been liquidated. Used furniture and medical equipment may not have much value in a liquidation, but accounts receivables tend to be a fairly robust asset and their liquidation often satisfies most, if not all, of the debt. Accounts receivables usually are valued for collateral purposes at 75% to 80% of balances outstanding less than 90 days, which provides the bank some collateral cushion in this worst-case scenario.

In the current debt market, most banks will agree to limit personal guarantees to several liability, but as noted above, often will insist that the several liability be increased from 100% of a pro rata share to a higher amount, such as 120% or 125%. This percentage is often negotiable.

OTHER FINANCING SOURCES AND METHODS

The availability of senior bank debt and low interest rates should not deter you from considering other viable and creative financing sources. Debt must be paid back out of future earnings and cash flow; some of the sources and methods below do not require repayment or they defer repayment, sometimes interest-free, into the future. The following sources and methods have a place in financing in certain situations.

Hospital Startup Feasibility Funding. As discussed in Chapter 1 and in more detail in Appendix A, hospitals in the later stages of what I call the "Cycle of Physician Employment" are often highly motivated to divest unprofitable physician practices. In such cases, the hospital may be willing to fund all or a portion of your startup feasibility in order to affect their divestiture as quickly as possible.

Hospitals' willingness to do this varies widely. As noted in Chapter 1, some hospitals will reject this as illegal out of hand, but in reality it isn't illegal, and we have seen it done many times. Paying for startup feasibility costs to affect an early termination in order to reduce future operating losses is a common business survival strategy. It is easily defensible from both a financial and legal perspective so long as the amounts paid are less than what the future losses would have been.

When broaching this subject with the hospital, remember that it works best when the hospital is at the point of urgently needing to rid itself of losses on employed physicians and when there is sufficient time left on your employment contract for them to realize a benefit from doing so. For example, if your employment agreement can be terminated with 180 days' notice or if it expires in 90 days and doesn't have to be renewed, there is little motivation or justification for the hospital to go down this path.

Physician Equity Investment. In the absence of hospital funding, an initial capital investment will be necessary to fund the legal and consulting fees to determine if a separation is possible and to complete the initial feasibility study discussed above. You likely will not be able to borrow to fund these costs because your group formation efforts are not far enough along—you haven't determined whether you can or should move forward with the group formation and no actual legal entity is in place to borrow funds from a bank.

In addition, banks like to see some level of equity investment in a business before they loan substantial amounts of money—otherwise known as "skin in the game." The theory is that you will be more engaged if you have something at risk up front. However, in the current environment, with senior debt financing readily available in many markets, we see banks requiring an equity investment only occasionally. Even the initial legal and consulting fees funded through personal investment often can be recouped by rolling them into the initial term loan for startup and soft costs once the decision has been made to proceed with the group formation. But remember what I told my daughter when she got her first credit card: debt is not money and *always* has to be repaid out of future earnings.

Note that the willingness to make an initial capital investment in legal and consulting fees to assess the feasibility of forming the group is a good way to gauge the actual commitment of your potential partners. My father always said, "talk is cheap until money is involved."

Private Healthcare Financial Firms. It is said that capital flows to business opportunities. A sure sign that a segment of physicians are seeking to reestablish private practices is that capital is flowing into private healthcare financial firms and is available specifically for that purpose. These companies specialize in financing physician projects such as practice startups as well as physician equity buy-ins to other healthcare entities, often without personal guarantees. One such company is Physicians Financial Partners (www.physiciansfp.com) based in Nashville, Tennessee.

Hospital Loan or Lease Financing. If you are repurchasing your furniture and equipment from the hospital, they might allow you to lease or financing the purchase through them. You normally would want to do this only if you find yourself reaching your debt capacity with the bank or if the bank lending market tightens because hospitals are legally required to charge market interest rates, and many are reluctant to loan money to physicians. However, if the hospital is motivated to terminate your employment or if debt capacity is an issue, this can be an option.

Physician Salary Deferral (Sweat Equity). Depending on the age and composition of the physicians forming the new group, simply foregoing your salary for the first few months after the group forms will reduce necessary borrowing dramatically.

If the hospital is willing to offer severance pay to terminate the contract early (discussed in Chapter 1) or where trailing bonuses or incentive payments are due from the hospital after your departure, these payments can be used to bridge this gap in salary.

Absent severance pay or trailing bonuses, a salary deferral would work only if a majority of the physicians have the personal financial resources necessary to go without a paycheck for several months, but it can be a viable option in some situations and should be considered.

Vendor Payment Terms. Many medical supply and drug vendors will offer 30- or even 45-day payment terms on purchases as an incentive to secure your business. This can dramatically reduce the level of borrowing required for working capital in the crucial early months of the practice, especially in specialties that need to maintain a large supply of drugs and injectables. Be cautious, however. Many of these vendors also offer discounts for early payment that you would be foregoing. Such discounts can be as high as 2%, and 2% per month is an effective borrowing cost of 24% per year. In such situations it clearly makes more sense to borrow the money from the bank and secure the discount.

Managing Payroll Dates. This may seem out of place on a list of financing sources, but it is actually an often-overlooked tactic that can lower or defer working capital borrowing needs in the crucial early months of a practice's operations. Practices typically pay staff every other week, so two months each year have three payroll dates. Simply establish the initial payroll date in such a way that the first month with three payroll dates is delayed as long as possible—preferably to the fifth or sixth month of operations. By that time, cash flow from the turnover of accounts receivable should be reaching normalized levels and the additional borrowing necessary to make that third payroll will be reduced or eliminated. Be careful to fully comply with any state or local laws, as some have limits on how often and when employees must be paid.

Pay-As-You-Go (PAYG) Practice Management Billing and Electronic Health Record Software. Another often-overlooked strategy to reduce upfront capital requirements and borrowing is to pay for software on a PAYG basis. Software typically is licensed, not sold, so you generally don't own it. Most software is updated regularly and the cost of such updates typically is included in your monthly software maintenance fees anyway. As a result, it makes less and less sense in today's environment to make a huge up-front capital investments in software with borrowed funds.

My company recently did a total cost comparison for a client of software vendors that offered practice management and EHR software, and found virtually no cost difference year over year between purchasing the licenses and paying for the subsequent upgrades through monthly maintenance fees compared to simply paying for the licenses on a monthly basis. Even ubiquitous software such as Microsoft Office and Adobe Photoshop are now routinely sold on a subscription or PAYG basis.

Assumption of Hospital Liabilities. Another source of financing that may seem out of place is the assumption of hospital liabilities. Why would you assume a hospital liability and what would it be?

A common liability of the hospital when a group leaves its employment is the liability for accrued vacation, sick pay, or paid time off of their employees who, in most situations, will become your employees after the separation. Hospital employee benefit policies generally require the employees be paid for their unused time off when their employment is terminated and they become your employees.

If you agree to assume this liability, the hospital will give you credit for the amount of the liability at closing, usually through a reduction of what you would otherwise owe them for the repurchase of your furniture, equipment, and other assets.

This liability doesn't cost you incremental cash. It is nothing more than agreeing to give those employees time off sometime in the future. Yes, you end up paying for it by paying the salary of those employees while they are not working, but those payments happen through your payroll process and occur over time and in the future. You likely would need to give those employees some sick time and vacation time during their first year of employment anyway. Assumption of this liability can be a beneficial way to reduce your borrowing.

A Third-Party Billing Company. The decision about whether to use a third-party billing company or do billing in-house needs to be carefully considered within the construct of your current situation. An outside billing company may make sense if the hospital has created a central billing office and your office lacks back-office billing staff. Hardware, practice management software, and EHR software decisions come into play here as well.

As a financing method, the benefit of a third-party billing company is that the company is paid only when the collections come in. So, the billing company is fronting the cost of the staffing and often all or a substantial portion of the software and hardware costs, while the cost to you is deferred until the cash is collected. While there are many other considerations in deciding between billing in-house or using an outside billing company, the upfront deferral of staffing costs and capital outlays needs to be part of this decision.

Ultimately the use of an outside billing company is a classic "make or buy" decision that should be considered and examined within the confines of your specific situation, but the added benefit of a one-time cost deferral in the crucial startup months should not be overlooked.

Equipment Leases. Equipment leases usually are the most expensive methods of acquiring medical equipment or furniture. Interest rates implicit in the leases often are two to three times the bank rates for a loan and, depending on the terms of the lease, you still may be required to purchase the equipment upon lease termination. In addition, leasing equipment generally means paying list price for the equipment. So while leasing can seem attractive, it usually isn't a good option so long as other financing options are available.

CHAPTER 5

Practice Startup, Operations, and Management

L et's face it: in the cottage industry that is small physician practices, a majority of the practices historically have not been well-run. That doesn't mean *all* practices are poorly run, but in starting a new group, or even a small solo or two-physician practice, you certainly don't want to be one of them.

Hiring an experienced practice manager or administrator is the single most important decision you will make at this point.

Recognize that in a startup, you are going to need someone who not only is experienced in running a practice, but someone who has the inimitable skills in *starting* a practice, too. That somewhat unique experience comes with a cost and skimping on what you are willing to pay for those skills and the skills of your other key staff is the worst mistake you can make.

As will be examined more closely in Chapter 6, during its critical first months of operations, any startup practice must be balanced precariously on what I call the three-legged stool. Two of those legs are held up by the practice manager or administrator and key staff you hire. My friend Michael Bouton, CEO of ViaTech Global, an employee assessment company based in Arizona (www.viatechglobal. com), says the chance of hiring the right person for a job based on the typical process of résumé reviews and in-person interviews is 50%.

You need to improve those odds. You don't have the leeway to make the wrong choice here.

Ultimately the success of your new business venture depends almost completely on being able to convert the gross charges generated by your practice of medicine into cash collections that will pay your overhead, repay your debt, and ultimately provide you a salary. Turning those charges into cash—the revenue cycle—coupled with managing costs, is key.

While there is a role for outside consultants here, engaging an outside consultant to complete the long list of tasks detailed in the checklist at the end of this chapter will be prohibitively expensive, and the results likely will be less than satisfactory. Operational implementation is best done by an experienced in-house full-time practice manager and key support staff with the oversight of an outside consulting resource.

Your practice manager will need to be hired and on board as an employee at least three months and preferably four to six months before your planned go-live date. This person will need to:

- Have a unique set of skills that go well beyond your typical practice manager;
- Share your vision or that of your physician partners;
- Be highly organized and experienced in group practice startups;
- Be capable of working closely with the physicians; and
- Be able to juggle the myriad tasks necessary to lay a strong foundation of business operations.

Your practice manager needs to be involved in virtually every decision concerning billing and collections, information technology, hiring, personnel policies, salary and wage rates, employee benefits, payor contracting, transfer of Medicare and other payor credentialing, and on and on.

No matter how qualified your practice manager is, however, you cannot cede responsibility for the ultimate decisions. The physician owner(s) and the practice manager must work together as a team. There has to be mutual trust and openness when problems arise. That said, the management style of the physician chosen to fill the role of physician leader must be one that establishes and maintains this level of trust.

As discussed in Chapter 1, if you are going to go down this road, you may be seeking to create a practice culture that is very different from that of your previous experiences in private practice. You must treat the practice manager with dignity and respect and fairly compensate him or her. You may need to increase the salary level in order to attract a candidate with the qualifications necessary to manage the practice and complete the tasks detailed in the checklist at the end of this chapter. Avoid the mistake of trying to hire someone on the cheap; to get the right person, you may need to prepare for "sticker shock."

Often the first candidate for your practice manager is your current manager under your hospital employment. This may or may not be a good choice. A careful assessment of the ability and willingness to put the time into the steps necessary for a successful startup, including complex information technology issues, payor contracting and credentialing, must be undertaken. Practice managers in large hospital-employed physician networks are generally used to myriad support resources in areas such as information technology, finance, accounting, billing, coding, and human resources. In a startup, at least initially, many of these responsibilities will fall on your manager.

Rarely will a manager have deep expertise in all areas. Don't hesitate to supplement the skills of your manager in areas where specific expertise is needed, such as information technology and finance.

STAFFING

Typically, the source for filling the other staffing roles in your new practice will be employees in your current office. While the hospital currently employs these staff members, they likely want you to offer them employment in your new group. This is another example of something that may need to be negotiated. While you are certainly under no obligation to offer these staff members employment, you probably will want a majority of the staff you have been working alongside on a day-to-day basis as part of your new practice.

Before approaching any staff members who are currently employed by the hospital, including any practice manager candidates, make sure you are permitted to do so. Many hospital employment agreements have a non-solicitation provision that prohibits soliciting staff. Be sure the legal discussions are far enough along and that you have the hospital's consent to approach the staff members if permission is required.

There may be current staff members you simply don't want working for you and there may be staff members who prefer to stay employed by the hospital. Salary and benefits also come into play here. Hospitals typically offer higher salaries and better employee benefits than most private practices. You may find that the salary levels of some of the staff members are higher than what fits into your budget. Employees will want to know what benefits you plan to offer and will have the expectation that their salary rates will stay the same, or even increase to offset any cuts in benefits.

If you do not plan to hire some of the staff and the hospital has a severance pay policy, the hospital may ask you to assume this obligation. While this may seem counterintuitive, remember that everything is part of a larger negotiation and this may not be an item worth fighting over.

At this stage, you are well on your way. The physicians and practice manager, together with the guidance of your advisors—attorneys, consultants, CPAs, and others—have the major of the pieces of the group in place. Now the hard work begins as you establish a target go-live date, continue legal negotiations, and work through the myriad operational tasks necessary for you to be ready to operate once again as a private practice.

Use this Practice Startup Checklist to guide you through the detailed steps of this process.

PRACTICE STARTUP CHECKLIST

1. Facility
- ❑ Sign lease agreement.
- ❑ Obtain signage.
- ❑ Arrange grounds and facility maintenance.

2. Legal
- ❑ Select local legal counsel.
- ❑ Determine entity type.
- ❑ Select practice name.
- ❑ Develop organizational documents.
- ❑ Obtain Federal Taxpayer ID.
- ❑ Obtain required state and local tax registration and permits.
- ❑ Obtain necessary business and occupational licenses.
- ❑ Initiate separation agreements with hospital.

3. Group
- ❑ Establish governance.
- ❑ Elect board and committees.
- ❑ Finalize pro forma.
- ❑ Establish startup budget and funding.
- ❑ Hire practice manager.

4. Accounting
- ❑ Select accounting firm.
- ❑ Establish accounts payable process.

❏ Establish budget and management reporting.

❏ Develop dashboards.

❏ Establish cash management process.

❏ Establish billing and accounts receivable process.

❏ Establish payroll processing system.

5. Banking Services

❏ Determine source of startup funds.

❏ Obtain line of credit.

❏ Determine signature authorization.

❏ Open checking account(s).

❏ Order checks, deposit slips, etc.

❏ Establish funds transfer procedures.

❏ Establish credit card processing.

6. Payor Enrollment/Contracting

  6.1. *Medicare*

  ❏ Contact MAC (Medicare intermediary) provider enrollment staff to confirm requirements, as they change and can vary.

  6.1.1. General steps:

  ❏ Apply for and obtain NPI for new group entity (required before any of the steps below). According to CMS, the timing can be as little as 10 days to receive the number.

  ❏ Complete Medicare form 855B for new entity.

  ❏ Complete Medicare form 855I (change of enrollment) for all providers.

  ❏ Complete Medicare forms 855R (reassignment) for all providers.

  ❏ Monitor enrollment status. Note: Enrollment status can be followed online using Enrollment Status Application Inquiry (ESAI) and should be monitored carefully.

6.2. *Commercial payors*

❏ Obtain carrier list from current system.

6.2.1. Contact provider contracting representatives for assistance and to confirm requirements for each payor.

❏ Confirm requirements for each payor.

❏ Will generally need the NPI for the new group before proceeding.

❏ The steps generally include completion of a provider change form for each provider.

❏ Additional contracting requirements and new payor contracts are likely for the new group.

  ❏ Obtain proposed contracts and fee schedules from each payor.

  ❏ Legal review

  ❏ Financial review

6.3. *Medicaid*

❏ Contact provider enrollment for specific requirements.

❏ Obtain NPI for new group prior to submission.

7. Equipment

❏ Review equipment valuations.

❏ Determine final equipment needs.

❏ Secure equipment financing/leases.

8. Insurance

❏ Secure general business insurance.

❏ Secure malpractice insurance.

❏ Secure business liability insurance.

❏ Secure workers comp insurance.

9. Personnel

- ❏ Review existing staff list and salaries.
- ❏ Determine which staff will be hired and salary rates.
- ❏ Establish employee benefit plans, including health insurance and paid time off policies.
- ❏ Establish employment policies and employee manual.
- ❏ Develop employment applications.
- ❏ Develop job descriptions.
- ❏ Develop policies for other HR functions, including hiring and termination.
- ❏ Establish payroll dates.

10. Office Services

- ❏ Provide referring physician listing for front desk.
- ❏ Establish telephone and phone number transfers.
- ❏ Hire answering service.
- ❏ Contract for Internet service.
- ❏ Establish domain name and email addresses.
- ❏ Secure cell phones/pagers.

11. Other Services

- ❏ Identify radiology services.
- ❏ Identify reference lab.
- ❏ Secure source for uniforms.
- ❏ Secure source for lab coats.
- ❏ Contract with laundry service.
- ❏ Contract for biohazard waste removal.
- ❏ Procure name tags.
- ❏ Contract for security system.

12. Marketing

- ❏ Have practice logo designed.
- ❏ Send out announcements.
- ❏ Hold an open house.
- ❏ Develop and print patient education brochures.
- ❏ Develop and print physician handouts.
- ❏ Place advertisement in Yellow Pages.
- ❏ Establish website and patient portal.
- ❏ Send marketing letters.
- ❏ Join Chamber of Commerce.

13. Compliance Issues

- ❏ Establish fire and safety inspection and fire evacuation plan.
- ❏ Obtain CLIA Certification.
- ❏ Undergo X-ray inspection.
- ❏ Secure OSHA training.
- ❏ Secure HIPPA training.
- ❏ Establish compliance training and compliance plan.

14. Billing and Collections

- ❏ Establish fee schedule.
- ❏ Establish patient financial policies.
- ❏ Develop scripts for reception, scheduling, and billing staff.
- ❏ Obtain allowable amounts from carriers.
- ❏ Develop encounter forms.
- ❏ Develop patient registration and medical history forms.
- ❏ Schedule staff training.
- ❏ Establish CareCredit relationship.
- ❏ Secure collection agency contract.

15. Manuals

- ❏ Policy and Procedures Manual
- ❏ HIPPA Compliance Manual and Wall Hangings
- ❏ OSHA Manual

16. Medical Records and Practice Management System

- ❏ Select system.
- ❏ Set vendor installation and training schedule.
- ❏ Oversee billing transition from hospital.
- ❏ Establish interim billing.

17. Miscellaneous

- ❏ Establish vendor relationships and payment terms.
- ❏ Secure petty cash/postage/change.
- ❏ Print stationery and envelopes.
- ❏ Print business cards.
- ❏ Other.

CHAPTER 6

Success Factors— Balancing the Three- Legged Stool

The risk of failure when starting an independent practice, even when you have an existing patient base, is greatest in the first year. Success requires balancing three key factors that will determine your ultimate survival:

1. Physician production: Your practice's ability to continue to generate gross charges at or above historical levels.
2. Revenue cycle management: The ability of your practice's management team to ensure those gross charges can be converted into cash collections in a timely manner.
3. Cost and overhead management. The ability of your practice's management team and outside accounting firm to monitor and manage overhead costs *as they are incurred*.

I refer to these three survival factors as the three-legged stool. A three-legged stool balances precariously, and if one leg doesn't hold up, the entire stool collapses. While collapse may not mean total failure, it likely means you will end up borrowing more than was planned. It might mean you reach your debt capacity with the bank and have to seek other sources of funds. It might mean you lack funds to pay overhead and have to cut staff hours or benefits or other costs. It might mean you have to reduce or go without a salary for a period of time.

While the three legs of the stool may seem pretty basic, during your first three to six months of operations, all three legs have potential weaknesses and are ripe for potential problems and failures. Even worse, in many cases you may not know it until it is too late. During the first three to six months of operations, the indicators typically used to measure the performance in these three key areas are either meaningless or unavailable. It's akin to driving blind in a snowstorm: You are unable to see where you are going and have few, if any, navigational aids to determine your speed, direction, or even if you are on your side of the road. The navigational indicators you normally would use don't exist in a meaningful form.

Let's look at each leg of the stool in more detail.

LEG ONE: MAINTAINING AND INCREASING PHYSICIAN PRODUCTION

Maintaining and increasing physician production is the best use of your time and effort and is the only leg of the three-legged stool that the physician owners can directly affect. Maintaining and increasing your production—doing the work, seeing the patients, putting in the time—is critical. While you may be able to compensate when other things go wrong in the revenue cycle as far as collecting the money from your production, lost production can never be made up.

If you are using a new electronic health record system and/or a different practice management system and implementing new and different work flows, it may be necessary to temporarily increase your workday, to work longer hours to keep up, to give up your regular day off, to work weekends. In short, you need to do everything you can to ensure production does not fall.

You don't have to maintain this new higher workload into perpetuity. Once you are sure the revenue cycle is functioning smoothly and cash collections are stable and overhead is coming in at reasonable levels, you can begin to go back to whatever you feel is a normal pace. But remember, medical practice is a fixed-cost business and the incremental cost of seeing an additional patient is almost nil. As a result, the revenue from that extra patient falls through to the bottom line.

Physician production is typically measured in private practices as either gross charges or cash collections.

Gross charges can be a good gauge of volume as long as the underlying fee schedule is consistent from period to period. However, now that you have returned to private practice, your standard fee schedule varies from what it was when you worked for the hospital. It may be higher or lower, but it is different and perhaps significantly different. So comparing historical gross charges to current gross charges probably will be meaningless.

In addition, your service mix—your mix of charges based on the types of services you provide—may have changed as well. The nature and extent of this will vary in each situation but say, for example, your practice provided x-rays while employed by the hospital. If you no longer provide that service, the gross charges won't be comparable.

Cash collections probably seem the most logical way to measure how you are doing in private practice. As one practice administrator notes, "I can't spend gross charges or work RVUs." The problem with cash collections should be even more obvious: you are starting with zero accounts receivable. As discussed in Chapter 3, it takes time for those receivables to turn over, and this accounts receivable ramp-up period means your cash collections in the first several months won't reflect normalized collection levels. Once the collections of the receivables stabilize after several months, you will have a fairly steady level of monthly cash collections. However, at this early stage, your cash collections have too many variables to be used as a navigational aid.

Since neither of these typical productivity indicators—gross charges and collections—is meaningful in a startup situation, there are two options available to measure production: patient visits and work relative value units.

Patient visits is by far the easiest way to measure your production level and ensure it is being maintained or increased. Review the data you have from your hospital employer about patient visits for a period of at least one year. Go back to your calendar and determine the number of days or half-day sessions you worked during that same time period and divide to come up with a "target" number of patients per day or per session. This should be your minimum goal and, preferably, you should increase this number by 5% to 15%.

Next, review your historical schedule template and determine if it needs to be revised to reflect your preferred practice style and if your available office work hours need to be increased to provide for additional capacity. Be sure to allow extra hours if you are learning a new EHR system. Then do everything you can to fill that schedule with patients. Consider, at least on a temporary basis, letting go or relaxing your scheduling "rules" by offering, if you don't already, same-day, early-morning, after-hours or weekend appointments. Remember, too, that patient no-shows may leave holes in your schedule, so don't be afraid to overbook and make sure your staff members are making reminder calls and confirming appointments on a consistent basis.

Keep a tick sheet of your patient visits count each day or session compared to your goal and monitor it to make sure you are meeting your target.

In specialty practices, patient visits may not be the indicator you need to track. Perhaps it is surgical cases or new consults or new OB patients or certain ancillary tests or procedures. Whatever your practice thrives on, set a goal and monitor your progress.

Work relative value units (wRVUs) have become familiar to most physicians leaving employment with hospitals because a majority of hospitals use them as the main component of their compensation plans.

While you may loathe wRVUs, they are the best way to measure production because they take into account both volume and work effort (coding)—the aspects of physician production. In addition, they are the underpinning of most physician reimbursement. For those who need a refresher in how wRVUs are developed and work, see Appendix B for a brief primer.

If your compensation under the hospital's employment was based in part on wRVUs, you should have easy access to historical data for comparison purposes, but it may need to be adjusted for any service mix changes as discussed above. They also may need to be adjusted for any modifiers you use.

Tracking wRVUs as you begin private practice may seem complex, but in most cases can be accomplished quite easily. Most physicians have 85% to 95% of their production in only 20 CPT codes. Have your practice manager, billing manager, or practice consultant create for you a grid listing these 20 or so CPT codes along with the wRVU value for each code. Simply track manually the number of times you bill each code and multiply that frequency by the wRVU value. Total your wRVUs for each day or week and compare to your historical productivity levels or goals. As with patient visits, your goal should be an increase in productivity levels of somewhere around 5% to 15% at least for the first few months.

The math here could easily be taken care of with a simple spreadsheet if you are so inclined. You may be tempted to have your practice manager or one of your staff maintain this for you but *resist that temptation.* This is *your* leg of the three-legged stool and is something in which you need to take personal ownership and focus. The job of your manager and staff is to hold up the other two legs; let them do the job you pay them for and don't distract them during this critical phase of your practice.

LEG TWO: REVENUE CYCLE MANAGEMENT

The revenue cycle encompasses all the processes and procedures that take place from the time a gross charge is generated until the payment is deposited in the bank.

Every time a patient is seen, a co-payment may be collected, posted to that patient's account, and deposited to the bank. A claim is filed with the insurance company for the services provided. The payor reviews the claim for completeness and pays you the contracted rate under the terms of your contract with them. The payment comes with an explanation of medical benefits, commonly referred to as an EOB, and is posted by your billing company or billing staff to each patient's account. Secondary insurance has to be filed in many cases, and many of the same process apply. Any remaining balance is billed to the patient.

If you see patients in the hospital, charges for those patients must be captured and entered too, along with charges for ancillary services, procedures, injections, supplies, drugs, and laboratory charges generated in your office.

All of this happens more than 100 times per week in a typical practice.

The revenue cycle, especially in the early stages of practice, is rife with potential problems. Most of the above processes are done electronically. Are the electronic claims going through to the payor? Have they been accepted? Do the payors have your new taxpayer ID number, group NPI number, and provider numbers? Have Medicare change of enrollment and reassignment of benefits been properly completed and have effective dates been confirmed? Is payor contracts information loaded properly in your practice management software? Are payments being spot checked against contracted amounts? Are claim rejections being followed up? Is patient insurance and demographic data being captured accurately and completely?

In short, is everything in place so payors can accept and process the claim? Establishing a relationship with your main commercial carriers' provider contracting representative and diligent follow-up are critical.

There can be additional complications if you installed and are using new practice management and billing software. Are staff properly trained on the system? Was it properly configured and installed? Were you able to "port" over the patient demographic information from the hospital's billing system or does your staff have to enter it for each patient? Are you transitioning to a new electronic health record and is that affecting your volume?

Any one or all of these issues can disrupt the revenue cycle, and without diligent, constant monitoring and follow-up on the part of your manager and staff, you may not know there are problems until the situation is critical from a cash-flow perspective. I can't tell you how many times I've heard the tale of how claims weren't going through to the payors and several weeks had passed before the practice discovered the problem.

Estimating your working capital needs and assuring you have sufficient borrowing capacity to have cash available to pay your overhead, salaries, and other expenses during the ramp-up period and to cover the downside if things go wrong is a critical part of the financial feasibility and financial projections developed in Chapter 3. The importance of making sure you have sufficient borrowing capacity for unexpected problems in your revenue cycle cannot be overemphasized.

If you've followed the advice offered in Chapter 5, you have identified and hired the best practice management and billing staff for your practice. You recognized that the skill sets in a practice startup situation are different than typical day-to-day practice management and operations. If your budget wouldn't allow you to hire staff with the experience in practice startups, I hope you've heeded my advice and supplemented that lack of experience with outside expertise.

Leg two of the stool is going to be held up solely by those choices you've made and you will need to trust them to successfully deal with the myriad potential issues that can go wrong in the revenue cycle.

While you will be busy holding up leg one by maintaining or increasing your productivity, you also need to ensure your management team and/or outside resources stay on top of these revenue cycle issues. Ask questions and get status updates about whether cash is being received and the level of outstanding accounts receivable. Lack of collections and ballooning accounts receivable balances are bad signs.

Here again, you are driving blind in a snowstorm. The pro forma monthly estimates of cash collections aren't reliable indicators of what should actually be coming in because there are so many variables to accurately apply them over short timeframes. The only thing that ultimately counts is collecting the money. When no EOBs are being received and payments being deposited, something is wrong.

Many physicians are afraid to go near the billing office and if that's the case with you, make sure somebody is getting status reports and closely monitoring the resolution of the inevitable issues that arise. You may also want to ask your practice CPA or consultant to monitor this on a weekly basis for the first several months.

LEG THREE: COST AND OVERHEAD MANAGEMENT

The other side of the cash flow equation is overhead. A detailed budget and pro forma should have been developed during the feasibility phase (Chapter 3). This budget should include estimates of one-time startup expenses and ongoing operating overhead.

Startup expenses and budgeted overhead during the first few months of operations tend to run higher than budgeted. As discussed in Chapter 3, pro formas and budgets done during the feasibility phase should be updated regularly as final decisions are reached on things such as staff salary levels, benefits, and other costs that were initially estimated.

Here, too, you are driving blind in a snowstorm. Income statements from your CPA will not be available until after the money is spent, so you will need to rely on your staff to monitor these expenses as costs are being incurred and bills are being paid. Have them identify as quickly as possible any problem areas or unanticipated costs.

Overhead percent, a common way practices measure and manage their overhead levels, will be a meaningless at this point. Overhead percent is the ratio of overhead to collections and collections, as discussed above, will be unreliable in the ramp-up mode and not meaningful until they have stabilized several months in the future. In addition, startup expenses and one-time costs that may not have been anticipated or accurately budgeted affect the other side of this ratio. Overhead percent likely will be a meaningless indicator during most of your first year of operations.

Most small practices (and many large ones) are not used to operating on a budget. Budget and overhead impacts from decisions such as staff raises, benefits, purchases, etc., tend to be looked at on a case-by-case basis as those decisions are made.

In smaller practices, the best way to manage overhead may be to simply sign all checks, or sign all checks over a certain nominal dollar amount and become aware of what is being spent where. Here again, you should avoid the temptation to micromanage because you need to be focused on production. A better approach is to manage by exception, making it clear that you want to approve any nonbudgeted expenditure over a certain dollar amount *before* it is incurred.

Payroll costs, which are usually the largest overhead expense in a practice, can also be managed by exception. Have your practice manager give you a comparison of actual payroll costs each pay period compared to budget, by individual employee if necessary.

Payroll costs tend to exceed budget as a result of overtime. If you've increased your office hours, you may need to stagger staff work hours to minimize or eliminate overtime. Establish a fairly strict overtime policy up front. Require office manager approval of any overtime and make sure the reason is documented. Sit down with the office manager each payroll period to discuss these reasons and work toward solutions that minimize or eliminate it.

Other expenses can be reviewed this way, too. The detail and quality of your financial and month cash flow projections are important here because they are the only indicator you'll have to compare to at this stage to gauge how you are doing.

Managing to balance the three-legged stool without the navigational aids that would typically be used to monitor performance can be precarious. Focusing on the above pathway will help get you through the first critical four to six months and lead to your ultimate success.

Epilogue

The obituary of the private physician practice has been written many times. I remember pronouncements that "the era of private practice is dead" going back more than 20 years. Physicians are trained to be independent thinkers and to function with a high degree of autonomy, and that may be why private practice has endured so long.

While the hospitals' success in this wave of employment has not been determined, warning signs of failure are appearing. I wonder about the financial sustainability of many of the hospital-employed physician networks already in place. Hospitals continue to consolidate, but bigger isn't always better and healthcare is still local. Will the "new money" arrive in time and in sufficient levels to sustain them? Are hospitals really the best partners to be at the forefront of integrated networks in the first place? Are they really the right organizational structure?

The cultural divide between younger and older physicians has been widening for many years, and this will continue to make it extremely challenging for physicians in private practice to recruit and sustain their business models as baby boomer physicians retire. I do not think private practice is dead, but I think it needs to evolve.

Some physicians, disillusioned with hospital employment, are terminating their employment and seeking to reestablish private practices. As I mentioned in the Introduction, I can't predict whether this trend will reach the level of "disintegration" that hospitals and physicians reached in the late 1990s, but the trend is irrefutably present. Clearly, many of these happy marriages are showing stress and aren't going to survive.

Many successful private physician groups continue to thrive in both single and multispecialty models, and maybe that tells us all we need to know. These physician practices can and will continue to survive over the coming years without being part of an integrated system. There will be many opportunities and options for them to participate in the new payment models as independent practices or they will create their own.

I hope this guide provided insight in evaluating these options and decisions. I use the word "important" many times throughout this guide and there are indeed many critical and "important" decisions to be made. I wish you success in both your decision making and in the direction you choose to go with your career and your livelihood.

There is no magic formula and there is no perfect model—success is in finding what works best for you.

The Cycle of Physician Employment

Those who fail to study history are doomed to repeat it.
ANONYMOUS

The 1990s saw a feeding frenzy of hospitals snapping up physician practices, paying huge acquisition prices, and guaranteeing the doctors cushy salaries. Within a few short years, hospitals were losing an average of $100,000 per physician annually and the acquisition binge became a divestiture binge. The resulting implosion was monumental. Long-tenured CEOs were dismissed, hospital debt ratings were lowered, and some hospitals had to be sold as a result of the huge losses sustained. Physicians found themselves having to reestablish themselves in private practice and facing the reality that their future incomes were going to decrease.

The trend of hospitals buying physician practices reemerged in the mid- to late-2000s as, once again, hospital acquisition and employment of physician practices became a common hospital strategy. At first, hospitals seemed more cautious, deliberately avoiding some of the strategies that had led to failure in the 1990s. Acquisition prices were generally void of goodwill and intangible asset purchases and compensation plans avoided guaranteed salaries, relying instead on productivity-based models.

This acquisition trend continues today, but the past few years have seen the reemergence of the transaction structures that led to the implosion in the 1990s: increasingly higher practice purchase prices (including intangible assets and, in some cases, goodwill) and higher compensation structures without concomitant productivity standards.

Has the reemergence of these two factors planted the seeds for another implosion?

The initial hospital strategy of acquiring and employing physicians to maintain or grow market share and assuring an adequate supply of physicians to support their mission has shifted. The post-Affordable Care Act (ACA) strategy is to develop the critical mass requisite for large, clinically integrated networks. Many hospitals believe these networks are necessary for participation in risk contracting, population health management, and accountable care payment models that government and commercial payors are attempting to establish.

As losses on employment of physicians mount, the question becomes twofold: 1) will the expected "new money" from these risk-based payment models and population health management arrive in time, and 2) will it be enough to sustain the losses? The jury is still out, but the losses represent an increasing risk to physicians looking to sell their practices as well as to the hospitals and health systems purchasing them.

AWARENESS AND ACTION

Physicians seeking to sell their practices and become hospital employees should make themselves aware that the hospital acquisition and employment of physicians seems to be repeating the cycle we saw in the 1990s. In its basic form, the cycle has three phases: Phase 1: Acquisition, Phase 2: Operational Development, and Phase 3: Restructuring/Divestiture. This cycle is illustrated in Figure 1.

Assessing where the local healthcare market or hospital is within this cycle can provide valuable insight to physicians who are considering returning to private practice, because it provides insight into likely future events.

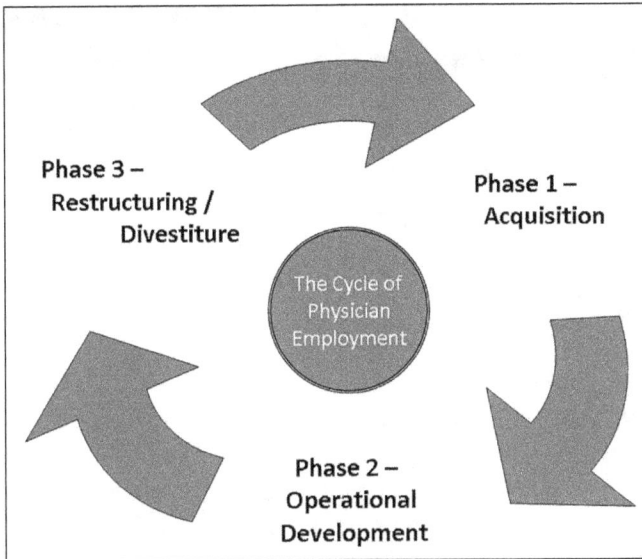

FIGURE 1. The Cycle of Physician Employment.

Signs indicate that this cycle, which went full circle in the 1990s, is doing so again and could be heading toward a collision course with economic reality. The Medical Group Management Association (MGMA) statistics on the median losses per physician for hospital/integrated delivery systems by specialty for 2014 and 2015 (2013 and 2014 data) are illustrated in Figure 2 (next page).

It is difficult to imagine that losses of this magnitude are sustainable. Moreover, the agencies that rate hospital bonds have long memories of the debacle that ensued in the 1990s. My company personally saw large and unceremonious waves of divestitures of physician practices as losses from physician employment mounted and borrowing costs were affected.

In addition, as noted above, it's not known whether "new money" will be injected into the reimbursement system and whether that money will benefit physicians. Many of these incentive payment systems are budget-neutral, meaning there will be winners and losers.

Specialty Net Loss Per FTE Physician*	2014	2015
Family Medicine	$192,213	$110,529
Internal Medicine	$249,339	$136,518
OB-GYN	$412,091	$252,635
Cardiology	$624,150	$388,260
Orthopedic Surgery	$356,582	$333,665
General Surgery	$465,184	$276,750
Average	$383,093	$249,726

FIGURE 2. The Medical Group Management Association statistics on the median losses per physician for hospital/integrated delivery systems by specialty for 2014 and 2015 (2013 and 2014 data). *Median loss excluding financial support per FTE physician for hospital/integrated delivery systems by specialty, 2014 data from the Medical Group Management Association 2014 Cost Survey for Single-Specialty Practices, 2015 data from Medical Group Management Association 2015 Cost and Revenue Report.

So far, the track record of the Pioneer Accountable Care Organizations (ACOs) for Medicare created under the ACA has been less than impressive. Of the 32 Pioneer ACOs that were created, one-third generated no savings at all and 70% of the savings that were generated were generated by three systems, all in the Boston area.

Perhaps even worse was the diminishing return from these initiatives; the savings in year two were half of the savings in year one, and downside risk hasn't even been factored into the equation yet. While many hospitals and hospital systems are "all-in" on this strategy, the question must be raised as to whether a hospital, which is inherently a huge cost center, is the logical place for elimination of unnecessary care, which is the cornerstone of these coordinated care and population health management initiatives.

Some hospital systems have or will figure it out, but many won't. It's a huge gamble. While hospitals expect to lose money employing physicians, as the cycle unfolds, they usually find the losses to be much higher than anticipated. This is often the result of failed implementation, the generous compensation offered to newly acquired employed physicians, and declining physician productivity. The need for additional management and information technology infrastructure emerges and, coupled with revenue cycle issues, the losses increase even more.

The "bet" is that the odds will change, that the new payment models will produce increased per-unit revenue. If that fails to materialize, and the initial indicators aren't good, the losses could quickly become unsustainable.

WHERE IS THE HOSPITAL INDUSTRY IN THIS CYCLE?

Most hospitals are somewhere in the late stages of Phase 2, the Operational Development Phase. While they may continue to acquire practices, most hospitals are struggling to evolve their operational and management infrastructure in order to realize cost efficiencies and to engage physician employees in governance.

Unfortunately, these activities—trying to gain cost efficiencies and engage physicians in governance—while necessary, aren't likely to solve the economic issues. In 30 years of working with physician practices I can say with certainty that the economic problems are unlikely to be solved on the operating cost side. The issues are almost always on the revenue side—provider productivity and the revenue cycle (billing, collections, payor contracts, and reimbursement rates)—or with the level of physician compensation itself.

While engaging physicians in governance is almost universally touted as a key tenet of a successful integrated network, the harsh reality is that this "governance," generally because of legal restrictions, usually comes with little or no authority. In fact, it is often no more than a feeble and transparent attempt to co-opt physician leadership to the hospital side in economic discussions. Rarely are physicians (or employees of any kind for that matter) willing or able to abide personal financial sacrifice for the good of an organization, no matter how much they are engaged in its operations. When was the last time you saw the CEO of a hospital agree to a 20% pay cut for the good of the organization?

In the later stages of Phase 2, the Operational Development Phase, the hospital begins to experience two other characteristics that inevitably lead to Phase 3, the Restructuring/Divestiture Phase: reorganization and "leakage."

Reorganization usually includes reshuffling or replacement of management and other changes in the organizational structure. During this stage, especially in large organizations, services such as staffing, IT, billing, and collections are outsourced to third parties. Consultants are brought in to assess the organization and a "redesign" of the compensation plan begins.

All of these efforts are driven by management's desire to "do something"—usually about the financial losses, although this is generally not explicitly stated. The management often uses the consultants' findings and compensation redesign as cover to try to affect changes—usually physician compensation changes (read "reductions")—that would not have been palatable in the earlier phases.

"Leakage" refers to the departure of physicians who, for whatever reason, have determined that employment with the network simply doesn't work for them. Naturally, the greatest motivation for physicians' departure is economic. Reductions in compensation are never palatable and whether such reductions are implemented under the guise of compensation plan redesign or simply happen because of preexisting contract terms or negotiation of new contracts doesn't matter. Economic motivation trumps. There are other reasons for physician departures, most notably the loss of control over the basic operation of the practice.

A notable generational difference arises here. Older physicians with prior experience in private practice are more likely to have issues with loss of control and the meetings and bureaucracy that come with being employed by larger organizations. Younger physicians are not as bothered by these things because their experience lacks perspective on the financial risk of private practice and the autonomy and responsibility that goes with it.

Knowing and understanding where the hospital or health system in your market is in this cycle is a key component if you previously sold your practice and are disenchanted and looking for other options such as a return to private practice.

While, as noted above, most hospitals are in the late stages of Phase 2, Operational Development, some have entered the early stages of Phase 3, Restructuring and Divestiture, whether they know it or not. Both my company and my (friendly) competitors are seeing leakage and a small but increasing number of unhappy physicians going back into independent practice. Paradoxically, some hospitals are in the early stages of Phase 1, Acquisition, and are just beginning to acquire and employ physician practices. It may be a few years before they reach the later stages of Phase 2.

Some hospitals have successful networks of employed physicians and a handful leaving to go back into private practice will not materially affect the viability of the network. Others may collapse from the sheer weight of the financial losses, CEO firings, bond rating declines, or from the mass departure of disillusioned physicians who have lost both confidence and interest in the business model.

It is said that healthcare is local and that is true. Each market is different, but a careful examination of the current situation in your market is in order. An accurate assessment of where your hospital is in this cycle will give you valuable insight into the future and aid you in both your decision-making and negotiating strategy.

The rest of this chapter provides a more detailed description of the characteristics of each phase of this cycle to further aid you in making this assessment.

PHASE 1—ACQUISITION

Hospitals enter into the acquisition and employment phase through many different paths. Some hospitals are forced into physician employment by the physicians themselves, as physicians seek income stability and shelter from day-to-day management responsibilities.

In other cases, physician employment is driven by the hospital's strategic planning process, which often includes a tenet to assure market access by establishing a strong and loyal primary care base. The ACA's provisions that encouraged development of ACOs led many hospitals to conclude that, strategically, they needed a network of physicians to clinically integrate in anticipation of these alternate payment models.

In still other cases, changes in Medicare reimbursement threatened the revenue base of many specialists, which led to a full-scale rush to "lock in" compensation at historical rates (or, more appropriately, historical rates plus a healthy increase) through hospital employment.

Whatever the motivation, Phase 1 is characterized by rapid acquisition, often with little time to give thought to development of the proper infrastructure to operate the employed practices. This is the phase where many mistakes are made that haunt the employed physician network for years to come and, in some cases, sow the seeds for its demise.

Physicians who are considering selling their practice to a hospital that is in this phase are in the "sweet spot" and rarely would a physician employed by a hospital in this phase be considering leaving.

PHASE 2—OPERATIONAL DEVELOPMENT

Phase 2 is generally characterized by evolving the operation of stand-alone physician offices to a more consolidated and standardized group practice platform. This sounds easy, but in reality often takes several years and overlaps dramatically with the late stages of Phase 1 acquisitions.

As the size of the network grows, the reliance on hospital services in areas such as human resources and finance becomes stressed. Usually a senior management position is created and filled by someone experienced in physician practice management. Power struggles between hospital and physician practice management are common and more often than not there is turnover at this position during the early years.

As losses become more apparent to hospital management and the hospital board, they often consider provider-based billing. In simple terms, provider-based billing allows the hospital to convert its employed physician offices to departments of the hospital for Medicare purposes. By meeting certain criteria, the hospital may bill Medicare under the Part A (the hospital side) for the facility fee component of, for example, an office visit, and Medicare Part B (the physician side) for the professional services of the physicians. While the reimbursement under Part B is reduced, the aggregate reimbursement increase is generally in the 20% range.

The downside is that patients now get two bills for a simple physician office visit and their out-of-pocket costs often increase, resulting in patient dissatisfaction and discontent—most of which is directed at the physicians and their office staff.

Another significant downside is that now part of every Medicare office visit must be billed using the hospital's billing system because the facility portion is billed and paid under Medicare Part A. These small charges are often quickly subsumed into the massive hospital billing system and, because of the relatively small dollar amounts involved, are difficult to track and evaluate from a collection standpoint. Measuring true performance on the actual collections on these charges is often impossible.

Commercial payors' handling of provider-based billing varies widely, depending on the state and the carrier. Some refuse to recognize this practice while others do, adding even more confusion to the mix.

In many cases, the shift to provider-based billing is a public relations nightmare for the hospital. We have seen some hospitals forced to reverse this practice in the face of community opposition and others avoid it altogether in anticipation of opposition. Sometimes, however, the shift to provider-based billing is implemented without incident. Many in the industry believe that federal budget pressures will ultimately lead to the reduction or outright elimination of provider-based billing and this will place even more pressure on hospitals already suffering under the weight of losses on employed physician practices.

As Phase 2 evolves, disparate operational processes are moved toward standardization and consolidation. Examples include billing, electronic health records, and financial reporting. Office site autonomy is further eroded as hospitals attempt staffing consolidation and cross-training and policies and procedures become more standardized. Additional infrastructure for information technology (IT) is often added. Benchmarking and financial reporting are standardized. Physician governance across the entire employed network is generally implemented.

As the accuracy of financial reporting and performance benchmarking are improved, most hospitals are unpleasantly surprised that operating losses are much higher than previously forecasted or reported. Such losses are almost always traceable to the revenue side of the equation: physician productivity and revenue cycle issues and the levels of physician compensation established through the acquisition negotiations in Phase 1. Physician productivity, once measurable, is often lower than anticipated, but the decline was often masked by inaccurate or incomplete data.

Basic billing and collection functions such as insurance verification, collection of copayments, and establishment and enforcement of patient financial policies, which are almost always lacking in the earlier stages, are shored up. Hospitals almost universally assert their payor contracts are superior to independent physician practices, but even this is generally found not to be the case.

While the losses are almost always traceable to the revenue side, hospitals usually focus on the cost side. Having failed to learn the old Tom Peters adage that your ability to cut overhead is limited but your ability to grow revenue is unlimited, hospitals generally focus on cutting costs.

The final step in Phase 2 is usually consolidation. Independent physician practices are generally run in a very cost-efficient manner. The same can't be said for hospitals. Generally the first step in hospital cost cutting is to combine previously cost-effective and efficient services at the practice level into a consolidated operating environment. This consolidation generally doesn't always include consolidation into one large physician office facility, but sometimes it does.

This consolidation step usually focuses on consolidation of business functions. My favorite is the central billing office or CBO. Consciously sending the people who know the patients to a CBO with an offsite location and phone number is a recipe for failure. In my 30 years in consulting with physician practices, I have rarely seen a CBO that improves collections or reduces costs—but that doesn't stop every hospital from trying. Another favorite of mine is consolidation of the scheduling function; the results are usually the same as with the CBO.

Phase 2 is where many independent-minded physicians begin to feel discontented and start to fantasize about regaining their independence.

PHASE 3—RESTRUCTURING AND DIVESTITURE

Phase 3 usually begins as a frenetic attempt to reduce operating losses and restructure the employed physician network into the viable long-term component of its business strategy. Hospitals rarely enter Phase 3 with the focus of divestiture, but that is sometimes the outcome.

The first step in the restructuring process usually involves bringing in an outside consultant to assess everything in the organization, from management to operations to strategy. The results of this assessment vary widely based on the situation. Sometimes it results in firing of the senior practice management team, which in some cases is warranted, but in many others is merely scapegoating.

Standardization of physician employment contracts, if not previously undertaken, is often tackled at this stage. In many situations, the term of the physician employment contracts are at or near their expiration anyway, and the expectation of reimbursement increases tied to non-productivity incentives as expected new payment models emerge opens the door for restructuring compensation.

We see intense effort being put into developing restructured compensation models in anticipation of population health management initiatives by payors. The problem is that, in most cases, these incentives haven't been defined. Most non-productivity incentives by payors involve "bonuses" from shared savings or for meeting certain coordination of care, outcomes, cost reductions, and compliance with evidence-based medicine guidelines.

One interesting sidelight to these "bonuses" or "new money" is an emerging debate over how it will actually be divided between the hospital and its employed physicians. The physicians assert they are the ones doing the extra work, changing their practice patterns, and (sometimes) foregoing productivity in order to meet these new guidelines and should therefore be entitled to the financial benefits.

Of course, the hospital perspective tends to be, although unspoken, that it is already subsidizing physician compensation and absorbing huge operating losses in developing the systems and technology supporting these new payor initiatives and it should be entitled to a substantial portion of this "new money" as a way to "pay back" or otherwise reduce the ongoing operating losses from the employed physician network.

Restructuring also can involve further consolidation of management services and revenue cycle functions, such as coding and billing as well as information technology. Previous consolidation undertaken in Phase 2 is often reconsidered, this time on a broader scale in the case of multi-hospital systems across a region or even an entire hospital system. This is usually done in the name of cost efficiency and standardization.

All of these efforts—assessment, management turnover, compensation restructuring, further changes in governance, and additional consolidation—are primarily motivated by a desire to do two things: reduce the level of losses from the employment of physicians and buy time.

At this stage, senior hospital management is usually under intense pressure from its governing board, the system corporate office or bond rating agencies, banks holding senior debt, or, in the case of publicly traded companies, Wall Street, to improve financial performance from employing physicians.

As this phase reaches its later stages, the result sometimes is a deliberate divestiture of underperforming practices or reductions in physician compensation that leave physicians looking for other options. Those physicians who are disgruntled enough begin to explore options and choose to try to make a go of it on their own by returning to independent private practice.

Often, leaving is not that simple. Leaving hospital employment and returning to private practice is often limited by contractual terms such as restrictive covenants and noncompete clauses. Depending on the specific contract terms, such departures may require the approval of the hospital employer, and such approval will likely preclude affiliation or sale to a competing hospital or large medical group. Divorces can get messy, and sometimes marriages last beyond their time because of such considerations.

Physicians interested in exploring independence at this stage in the cycle may find the navigation of any legal and financial hurdles easier.

The hospital's drive to dramatically reduce losses removes barriers to departure fairly quickly. In the late 1990s, for example, we saw some hospital systems virtually give the physicians back their practices. In some cases, hospitals paid physicians severance to terminate their contracts early and paid for consulting fees to support the physicians going back on their own—all in the interest of getting the losses off their books as soon as possible.

A final interesting sidelight of physicians returning to private practice is that hospitals almost always try to keep such departures as low profile as possible—almost as though they fear that widespread knowledge of disgruntled physicians leaving will create a stampede for the door. Based on what happened last time the industry experienced this cycle, you can't help but wonder if the time will come when hospitals will welcome that stampede.

WHERE DOES THIS LEAVE US?

Is the cycle described above the fate of every hospital system that employs physicians? No. Some hospitals and hospital systems have and will continue to have long-tenured, successful physician employment models. New or fresh models for successful networks may emerge. They have or will figure it out. Others, as also noted, are just getting started and their history hasn't been written.

Determining where your hospital is in this cycle and assessing its ability to attain and retain success is key. The outline above and the checklist at the end of this appendix can provide insight to help you make this judgment in your market situation.

THE CYCLE OF PHYSICIAN EMPLOYMENT ASSESSMENT CHECKLIST

Check the traits currently present in the hospital's employed physician network in each phase listed below. Generally, the area where you stop making checkmarks will indicate the phase in which your hospital is currently operating its employed physician network and how far it is into that phase.

In general, the farther a hospital is into this cycle, the more malleable they will be to a physician seeking to leave employment and return to independent practice.

Phase 1—Acquisition

❑ No formal or communicated acquisition/employment strategy
❑ Few employed physicians
❑ Little or no experience in employing physicians
❑ Flexibility and wide variances in compensation and employment contract terms
❑ Little or no physician practice management infrastructure
❑ Little or no physician engagement in governance
❑ Multiple billing systems at practice level
❑ Hospital departments providing services such as finance, HR, IT

Phase 2—Operational Development

❑ Base of employed physicians (non-hospital based) with at least 1–3 years tenure
❑ Consolidation of billing and EHR onto common software platform
❑ Hiring or presence of senior physician practice management personnel
❑ Implementation of or functioning physician governance
❑ Implementation or moving toward operational standardization
❑ Moving toward standardization of physician compensation model

❏ Little flexibility in contract terms—standardization of employment contracts
❏ Staffing consolidation and cross-training
❏ Centralization of operating functions such as billing
❏ Network operating costs being allocated to practice level

Phase 3—Restructuring and Divestiture
❏ Concerns expressed on operating losses of physician practices
❏ Outside consultants engaged in practice assessments and performance improvement
❏ Turnaround plans or performance improvement plans
❏ Compensation plan restructuring
❏ Turnover of physician practice management
❏ Use of interim or outside physician practice management
❏ Bond rating downgrades
❏ Hospital C-suite turnover
❏ Physicians leaving the network to return to private practice—"leakage"
❏ Outsourcing of operating functions such as billing and non-clinical staffing
❏ Consolidation of operating functions at corporate or system-wide level.

Work RVU Primer

R elative Value Units (RVUs) are part of the resource-based relative value scale (RBRVS) that transitioned to a standardized Medicare physician payment method in 1992.

Work RVUs (wRVUs) are assigned to each procedure performed by healthcare providers. As the name implies, wRVUs measure *work* effort of one procedure relative to another. Specifically, wRVUs take into account the following:

- Physician time required to perform the service;
- Technical skill and physical effort;
- Mental effort and judgment; and
- Psychological stress associated with physician's concern about the risk to the patient.

Perhaps the easiest way for physicians to think of wRVUs is to think of one of the most commonly used CPT codes 99213—Office/outpatient visit, established patient level 3—as 1 wRVU (actually, it is .97 wRVU). Contrast that with CPT code 99214—Office/outpatient visit, established patient level 4—at 1.5 wRVU, and you start to understand how it works.

Since the government is involved, naturally it isn't as simple as it sounds. For one thing, wRVU values can and do change periodically and such changes are generally required to be revenue neutral to Medicare. So if one CPT code's wRVU value goes up, others will go down.

There are two other types of RVUs: practice expense (PE) and malpractice (MP). These two types are adjusted for geographic cost factors to reflect local or regional variances in operating expenses and the risk of malpractice claims inherent in individual CPT codes.

The total of these three RVUs (work, PE, and MP) are multiplied by a national conversion factor to arrive at the allowable payment amount for the Medicare physician fee schedule.

The beauty of wRVUs is that they are universal across all specialties and geographic regions. So if you can determine your wRVUs, which as noted above inherently take into account both your volume of work effort and your coding, it becomes easy to compare your productivity with that of other physicians in your specialty on a national basis. This universal ability to compare physicians is why hospitals rely on them so much.

How do you determine your wRVUs? wRVU values for each CPT code are published at least annually as part of the Medicare Physician Fee Schedule and are available at the Centers for Medicare & Medicaid Services (CMS) Web site at www.cms. gov/physicianfeesched/pfsrvf/list.asp as well as at many other Internet sites. Care must be taken if you or your office manager undertake this effort manually, however, as raw wRVUs often need to be adjusted based on use of CPT code modifiers. Your practice consultant may need to help you with these adjustments if you use a lot of modifiers in your specialty.

Many newer practice management software packages also provide wRVU data, although I urge caution here, too. As noted above, wRVU values can and do change, so you want to be sure your software provider has updated the values in your system. Outdated wRVU values in practice billing systems is, in my experience, the rule rather than the exception.

There are many other resources that can cost effectively determine your wRVUs. One resource I like is the InfoDive® tool offered by Trellis Healthcare (www.trellishc.com).

There are other pitfalls in ensuring that you have accurate wRVU data. For example, if your practice uses mid-level providers such as physician assistants or nurse practitioners, you want to make sure you are not counting their wRVUs for services billed under your name ("incident to") as part of your productivity.

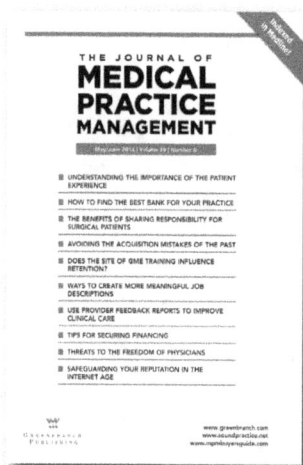

www.ingramcontent.com/pod-product-compliance
Lightning Source LLC
Chambersburg PA
CBHW061611220326
41598CB00024BC/3543